BREATHE TO HEAL

BREAK FREE FROM ASTHMA

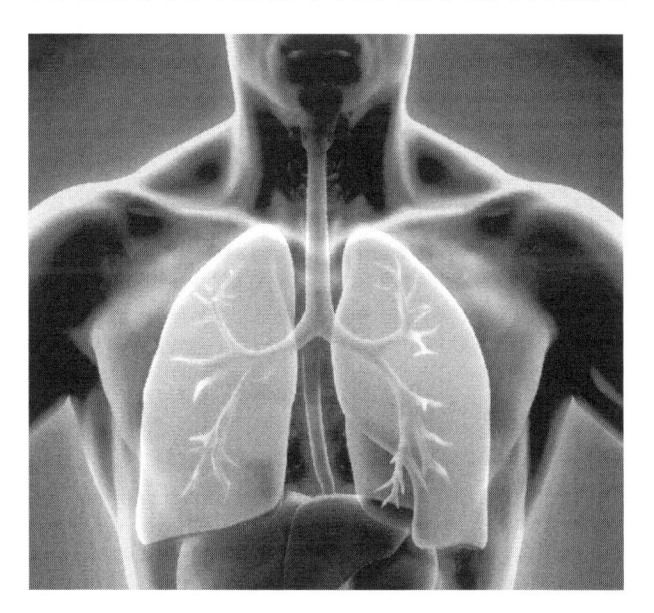

SASHA YAKOVLEVA

K.P. BUTEYKO, MD-PhD, A.E. NOVOZHILOV, MD

THOSE WHO TAMED THEIR ASTHMA

Breathe To Heal
Copyright © Breathing Center
All Rights Reserved

No part of this book may be reproduced or utilized in any form or by any means, including photographs, recordings, or by any information storage or retrieval system or technologies now known or later developed, electronic or mechanical, without permission in writing from the publisher, Breathing Center LLC. **www.BreathingCenter.com**

ISBN: 978-1537126609

Printed in the USA

Disclaimer:
This book is presented solely for educational purposes. It is not intended as a substitute for the medical advice of a health professional. The reader should regularly consult a physician in matters relating to his/her health and particularly with respect to any symptoms that may require diagnosis or medical attention. The publisher and authors are not responsible for any specific health needs that may require medical supervision and are not liable for any damages or negative consequences from any treatment, action, application or preparation to any person reading or following the information in this book. Any use of the information in this book is at the reader's discretion. The authors and the publisher specifically disclaim any and all liability arising directly or indirectly from the use or application of any information or instructions contained in this book.

Written by: S. Yakovleva; K. Buteyko; A. Novozhilov; and those who tamed their asthma
Illustrations: Victor Lunn-Rockliffe, Arash Akhgari
Forward: Thomas Fredricksen
Intro article: Jane E. Brody
Book interior design by Jean Boles
Cover design by Matra Communications
Illustration on the cover: © Nerthuz

TABLE OF CONTENTS

ACKNOWLEDGEMENT
by *Sasha Yakovleva* 10

SECTION 1:
INTRODUCTION
A Breathing Technique Offers Help for People With Asthma
by *Jane E. Brody, The New York Times* 12

Foreword by *Thomas Fredricksen* 17

SECTION 2:
UNDERSTANDING OVER-BREATHING
by *Sasha Yakovleva*
Asthma: The Conventional Treatment Versus The Buteyko Therapy 26

Hyperventilation and its Ramifications, Including Asthma 38

Biography of K.P. Buteyko, MD-PhD 48

About A. E. Novozhilov, MD 58

SECTION 3:
THE MEDICINE OF THE FUTURE
by *Konstantin P. Buteyko, Md-Phd*
About Asthma..61

The Theory of My Method..63

List of Health Problems Triggered by Hyperventilation.........67

SECTION 4:
BUTEYKO BREATHING MANUAL
by *Andrey Novozhilov, MD*

    Part 1: Buteyko Theory 72

        Introduction 72

- Theoretical Basis 73
- Asthma—A Defense Mechanism 74
- The Hyperventilation Provocation Test 75
- The Development of Asthma and Conventional Therapy 76
- CO2 Levels in the Lungs and in the Blood 76

Part 2: Breathing Awareness and Measurements 83
- Mindfulness of Breathing 83
- Breathing 83
- Various Breathing Measurements 86
  - 1. Control Pause 86
  - 2. Positive Maximum Pause 86
  - 3. Negative Maximum Pause (or Absolute Maximum Pause) 87
- About Control Pause 87
  - How to measure Control Pause 88
  - The most important thing to remember 89
  - The Morning Control Pause 89

Part 3: Buteyko Breathing Exercises 91
- Understand How To Do The Exercises 91
- When and for how long you should do the Buteyko breathing exercises? 93
- What to do if you are not experiencing symptoms? 94
- Consult your Breathing Normalization Specialist 94
- How can you tell that you are doing the exercises correctly? 96
- Choice of Exercise 96
- Key points about breath-holds 97

Exercise # 1: How to reduce the volume of breathing through relaxation 98

    Approach 1: Awareness of the breathing process...............99

    Approach 2: Extraordinary sense of well-being 101

    Approach 3: Just hint at reduction of airflow 103

    Notes for Exercise 1 – Approach 1, 2 and 3 (*Possible mistakes*)..104

Exercise # 2: Holding your breath 106

    Possible Mistakes...108

Exercise # 3: Holding Your Breath During Physical Exercise.....108

    Possible Mistakes...110

Exercise # 4: Many short breath-holds throughout the day.....111

    Possible Mistakes...111

    Important rules for all Buteyko breathing exercises 111

    Caution...112

Emergency Exercises to Combat Asthma Attack 113

    Emergency exercise 1 – Many small breath-holds 113

    Emergency exercise 2 - Relaxation instead of exhalation..114

    Emergency exercise 3 - Relaxation during the exhalation .116

Exercises to Stop Symptoms 116

    1. Unblock your Stuffy Nose 116

    2. How to stop coughing...117

    3. Sneezing 117

    4. How to use physical exercise to control asthma symptoms...118

Part 4: Lifestyle Instructions..120

    Cleansing reactions 120

How to prevent hyperventilation during sleep 121

How to prevent hyperventilation when speaking 122

Buteyko and diet.. 122

How to keep motivated to practice the Exercises 123

Part 5: Use of Steroids for Asthma 124

Buteyko's quick and safe steroid course for asthma 124

Principles... 127

What types of steroids are suitable?.............................. 129

When to take steroids... 129

Protocol for steroid therapy in the Buteyko treatment of asthma 132

How to determine if the dose is correct (neither excessive nor insufficient) 133

Dose reduction and termination of steroid therapy.......... 138

How long do you need to take steroids? 138

SECTION 5:
BREATHING NORMALIZATION FOR CHILDREN
by *Sasha Yakovleva*

Part 1: Breathing and its Measurements 143

Over Breathing 143

Healthy Breathing 144

Close Your Mouth 144

Why does my child hyperventilate? 146

Breathing Measurements... 147

How to take breathing measurements............................... 148

When to take breathing measurements.............................. 151

How to record breathing measurements 152

How to read breathing measurements	152
Healing Crisis	156
Part 2: Lifestyle Recommendations	**159**
Stress Reduction	159
Breathing During Sleep	160
Tape	161
Scarf	162
Other factors	163
Physical Activity	163
Diet	165
What to drink	165
What to Eat	165
Hunger	167
Salt	167
Nature	168
Talking	169
Part 3: Breathing Exercises for Children	**171**
I. Breathing Exercises in a Still Position	175
1. Do I Breathe Through my Mouth?	175
2. American Indian Mother	176
3. Show Me Your Breathing	177
4. Are my Shoulders/Chest/Stomach Moving?	178
5. Is my Breathing Noisy?	179
6. Book on the Belly	180
7. Hug a Tree	180
8. A little Mouse.	181

- 9. Be a Samurai..181
- 10. Tape Exercises..182
- 11. Nose Songs...184
- 12. Polly's Angel...185
- 13. A Sophisticated Device 185
- 14. Fixed Breath Holds 187
- 15. Flexible Breath Holds..187

II. Breathing Exercises in Motion 188

- 16. Airplane 189
- 17. Dancing with a Nose Song..189
- 18. Walking, Hiking, Running 190
- 19. Don't Miss the Fridge..192
- 20. A Corner-to-Corner Walk with Breath Holds 192
- 21. Steps with Breath Holds 193
- 22. Walk with Breath Holds 194
- 23. Simple Jumps 194
- 24. Three-Fold Jumps 195

III. Breathing Exercises for Relaxation 198

- 25. Imagine..199
- 26. I am Not a Robot 200
- 27. Heating Pad...201
- 28. Tense Up 201

IV. Breathing Exercises to Stop Symptoms 202

- 29. Nodding 202
- 30. The Breathing Guru 203
- 31. Coughing...204

SECTION 6:
THE LIVING MIRACLE

Part 1: Testimonials by *People Who Tamed Asthma* 206

Part 2: Questions And Answers About Asthma 248

Part 3: Breathing Normalization Products And Services 265
    DVD and Downloads 265

    CDs and Downloads 266

    Books and Downloads 267

    Educational Services Online 268

AFTERWORD
Help Others Learn About Dr. Buteyko's Breathing Normalization by *Sasha Yakovleva* and *Thomas Fredricksen* 270

ACKNOWLEDGEMENT

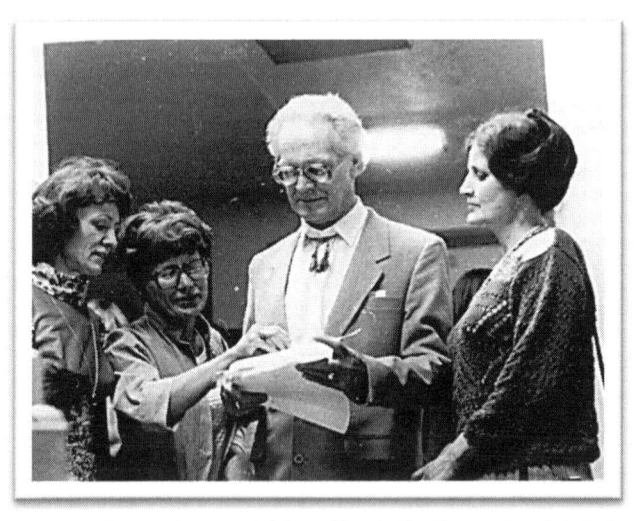

K.P. Buteyko and his wife, L.D. Buteyko (right), with their students

I believe this book began taking shape in 1952 in Moscow during one of the nights when Dr. Buteyko was alone in a room in the hospital where he worked. He was standing in front of a window contemplating the question, "Why do people get ill?" At this moment, a bright flash of light forced him to lower his gaze and notice that his torso was moving driven by his heavy breathing. This was the moment when Dr. Buteyko realized that over-breathing could act as a trigger for asthma and other health problems. Since then, his work has been continuously helping people, primarily asthmatics, to heal—first in the Soviet Union, then all over the world. Without these people who managed to overcome their health challenges by reducing their breathing, this book would be impossible. And of course, it also would be inconceivable without Dr. Buteyko's wife and kindred spirit— Ludmila Buteyko, the mother of Andrey E. Novozhilov, MD. Both, Ludmila and Andrey, have dedicated their lives to preserving this miracle-like method for future generations. I thank you all!

- Sasha Yakovleva

SECTION 1: INTRODUCTION

By Jane E. Brody, *The New York Times*

Foreword by Thomas Fredricksen

A Breathing Technique Offers Help for People With Asthma by *Jane E. Brody, The New York Times*

The New York Times

In 2009, The New York Times published an article about the work of the Breathing Center (formerly Buteyko Center USA) regarding asthma. This article was written by Jane E. Brody, the Personal Health columnist for The New York Times; the article became extremely popular and instantly made the word "Buteyko" well known all over the world. It helped many asthmatics to find the Breathing Center and receive help they critically needed. With the permission of The New York Times and Jane E. Brody, the text of this legendary article is published below.

I don't often write about alternative remedies for serious medical conditions. Most have little more than anecdotal support, and few have been found effective in well-designed clinical trials. Such trials randomly assign patients to one or two or more treatments and, wherever possible, access the results without telling either the patients or evaluators who received which treatment.

Now, however, in describing an alternative treatment for asthma that does not yet have top clinical ratings in this country (although it is taught in Russian medical schools and covered by insurance in Australia), I am going beyond my usually stringent research criteria for three reasons:

The treatment, a breathing technique discovered half a century ago, is harmless if practiced as directed with a well-trained therapist.

It has the potential to improve the health and quality of life of many people with asthma, while saving health care dollars.

I've seen it work miraculously well for a friend who had little choice but to stop using the steroid medications that were keeping him alive.

My friend, David Wiebe, 58, of Woodstock, N.Y., is a well-known maker of violins and cellos, with a 48-year history of severe asthma that was treated with bronchodilators and steroids for two decades. Ten years ago, Mr. Wiebe noticed gradually worsening vision problems, eventually diagnosed as a form of macular degeneration caused by the steroids. Two leading retina specialists told him to stop using the drugs if he wanted to preserve his sight.

He did, and endured several terrifying trips to the emergency room when asthma attacks raged out of control and forced him to resume steroids temporarily to stay alive.

Nothing else he tried seemed to work. "After having a really poor couple of years with significantly reduced quality of life and performance at work," he told me, "I was ready to give up my eyesight and go back on steroids just so I could breathe better."

Treatment from the '50s

Then, last spring, someone told him about the Buteyko method, a shallow-breathing technique developed in 1952 by a Russian doctor, Konstantin Buteyko. Mr. Wiebe watched a video demonstration on YouTube and mimicked the instructions shown.

"I could actually feel my airways relax and open," he recalled. "This was impressive. Two of the participants on the video were basically incapacitated by their asthma and on disability leave from their jobs. They each admitted that keeping up with the exercises was difficult but said they had been able to cut back on their medications by about 75 percent and their quality of life was gradually returning."

A further search uncovered the Buteyko Center USA in his hometown, newly established as the official North American representative of the Buteyko Clinic in Moscow.

"When I came to the Center, I was without hope," Mr. Wiebe said. "I was using my rescue inhaler 20 or more times in a 24-hour period. If I was exposed to any kind of irritant or allergen, I could easily get a reaction that jeopardized my existence and forced me to go back on steroids to save my life. I was a mess."

But three months later, after a series of lessons and refresher sessions in shallow breathing, he said, "I am using less than one puff of the inhaler each day—no drugs, just breathing exercises."

Mr. Wiebe doesn't claim to be cured, though he believes this could eventually happen if he remains diligent about the exercises. But he said: "My quality of life has improved beyond my expectations. It's very exciting and amazing. More people should know about this."

Ordinarily, during an asthma attack, people panic and breathe quickly and as deeply as they can, blowing off more and more carbon dioxide. Breathing rate is controlled not by the amount of oxygen in the blood but by the amount of carbon dioxide, the gas that regulates the acid-base level of the blood.

Dr. Buteyko concluded that hyperventilation—breathing too fast and too deeply—could be the underlying cause of asthma, making it worse by lowering the level of carbon dioxide in the blood so much that the airways constrict to conserve it.

This technique may seem counterintuitive: when short of breath or overly stressed, instead of taking a deep breath, the Buteyko method instructs people to breathe shallowly and slowly through the nose, breaking the vicious circle of rapid, gasping breaths, airway constriction and increase wheezing.

The shallow breathing aspect intrigued me because I had discovered its benefits during my daily lap swims. I noticed that swimmers who had to stop to catch their breath after a few lengths of the pool were taking deep breaths every other stroke, whereas I take in small puffs of air after several strokes and go indefinitely without becoming winded.

The Buteyko practitioners in Woodstock, Sasha and Thomas Yakovlev-Fredricksen, were trained in Moscow by Dr. Andrey Novozhilov, a Buteyko disciple. Their treatment involves two courses of five sessions each: one in breathing technique and the other in lifestyle management. The breathing exercises gradually enable clients to lengthen the time between breaths. Mr. Wiebe, for example, can now take a breath after more than 10 seconds instead of just 2 while at rest.

Responses May Vary

His board-certified pulmonologist, Dr. Marie C. Lingat, told me: "Based on objective data, his breathing has improved since April even without steroids. The goal now is to make sure he maintains the improvement. The Buteyko method works for him, but that doesn't mean everyone who has asthma would respond in the same way."

In an interview, Mrs. Yakovlev-Fredricksen said, "People don't realize that too much air can be harmful to health. Almost every asthmatic breathes through his mouth and takes deep, forceful inhalations that trigger a bronchospasm, 'the hallmark of asthma.'"

"We teach them to inhale through the nose, even when they speak and when they sleep, so they don't lose too much carbon dioxide," she added.

At the Woodstock center, clients are also taught how to deal with stress and how to exercise without hyperventilating and to avoid foods that in some people can provoke an asthma attack.

The practitioners emphasize that Buteyko clients are never told to stop their medications, though In controlled clinical trials in Australia and elsewhere, most have been able to reduce their dependence on drugs significantly. The various trials, including a British study of 384 patients, have found that, on average, these who are diligent about practicing Buteyko breathing can expect a 90 percent reduction in the use of rescue inhaler and a 50 percent reduction in the need for steroids within three to six months.

The New York Times Article by Jane E. Brody

The British Thoracic Society has given the technique a "B" rating, meaning that positive results of the trials are likely to have come from the Buteyko method and not some other factor. Now, perhaps, it is time for the pharmaceutical supported American medical community to explore this nondrug technique as well.

By *Jane E. Brody*

From The New York Times, November 3, 2009 © The New York Times. All rights reserved. Used by permission and protected by the Copyright Laws of the United States. The printing, copying, redistribution, or retransmission of this Content without express written permission is prohibited.

Foreword by Thomas Fredricksen

Thomas Fredricksen is a psychologist, co-founder of BreathingCenter.com and Advanced Breathing Normalization Specialist. At the age of fifty-five, he became an invalid due to a sudden upsurge of his asthma. The Buteyko Method saved his life and showed him the way to help people improve their breathing and health.

My Nightmare

For many months, night after night, I had a recurring nightmare: I am standing by the door to my house as if I am going somewhere or waiting for someone. My heart is racing out of control. I am grasping for breath. My lungs feel as if I am suffocating, but I cannot exhale. My mind is in total panic. I turn to my wife, Sasha, who asks me again and again if she should call 911. I say, "No," though I know I should say "yes."

My Reality

I would then wake up in my bed, gasping for air and in ultimate fear. The fear would hit me because this nightmare was my reality. It was not a bad dream—it was my life. The worst part was that there was nothing at all I could do about it.

The coughing fits and episodes of near suffocation made my life a living hell. Most nights, I coughed for many hours at a time, praying for it to stop, and being more frightened than I have ever been in my life. Eventually it would stop, and for a reason that still doesn't make sense to me, I would then feel safe. I must have thought it would never happen again, though that thought was not at all rational because the coughing would come back the next time I slept, the next time I went out into the cold, got too close to our dog, or tried to do any physical work or exercise. Almost anything could trigger the attack, even feeling stressed, which was an all-too-common experience at that point.

Foreword by Thomas Fredricksen

My Story

In 1978, I became sick with Legionnaire's disease, which turned into a severe case of pneumonia. Although many people die from this illness, I survived. When it was over, the doctors said my lungs had been damaged and that I would be asthmatic for the rest of my life.

I was still in my twenties and soon felt healthy again. Once in a while, a flu or cold would cause my breathing to sound raspy. If it was particularly bad, I'd use a rescue inhaler, which would clear everything up and I would forget all about it. I would throw the inhaler into a kitchen drawer or a glove compartment, and it would be left there until I became sick again in a year or two. I moved through my adult life as an active, energetic person. I achieved the rank of Black Belt in American Karate. I lifted weights and ran in competitions. I swam and surfed and "played hard." I had mild asthma—"So what?" I thought. I accepted my inhaler as a necessary part of life. I got a little worse each year, but after all, I was getting older.

In 2007, when I suddenly became sick with a severe flu, I wasn't surprised when I needed to use an inhaler. My doctor also recommended that I take a course of antibiotics. When the flu continued and I needed a second dose, I thought nothing of it. Another dose would help me get on with my life, or so I thought... but I did not completely recover. Instead, I routinely became breathless and continued to feel as if I was suffocating.

My doctor then recommended a stronger rescue inhaler. I agreed, expecting it to cure me. I also took all the medication that was now prescribed to me. Then, I was told that I had to take steroids. What followed next was a prescription for the stomach problems caused by the steroids. And then the dosages of all medications were increased.

I had heard of all these medicines before. Who hasn't? It seems that every third commercial on television is about a new medication for breathing difficulties. On the screen are happy people, walking, dancing, or playing with kids. When the actors speak, they talk of the freedom they've found. "Just take your medicine, and you'll be fine!" is their message to everyone.

I was not fine. At the beginning of the nightly attacks, these treatments provided some relief—at least for a couple of hours. As time went on, however, these moments of forced relief became very rare, until my rescue inhaler seemed to actually worsen the condition. I know my doctors and the pharmaceutical companies were doing their best, but unfortunately, that was not good enough; my symptoms only increased. I wondered if this illness, which already ruled my life, would be the death of me.

I felt as if something was not quite right with the whole logic of my treatment. My body was treated like a broken machine that produced unwanted symptoms. The doctors were comparable to army generals, who kept coming up with new tactics. Under their supervision I would go to a pharmacy, buy the best available weapons and fight against my symptoms. We were all trying hard, but the war wasn't ending. Listening to the same TV commercials again and again, I became more aware of the voiceover warning people of endless side effects, including potential fatality, which these "miracle drugs" could cause.

Meanwhile, my illness became a part of our life. In some ways, it seems you get used to anything if it happens long enough. My family started rotating their lives around my asthma. Everything we did or did not do was dictated by how I felt. My wife's experience with my illness was, in many ways, worse than mine. She was constantly trying to find something to help me, some home remedy that would provide, at least, a relief. I tried everything, hoping that something would finally work and make us both feel better. At night, I tried to hide my struggles. Of course, the moment Sasha realized I wasn't in bed next to her she would search the house, filled with the fearful thought that she would find me too late.

Even now, as I recall this story, I strongly feel the pain and frustration of those times. I am also reminded of why, today, all my efforts are directed toward not only sharing the story of my suffering, but more importantly, the story of my success—my freedom from breathing difficulties.

The Cure

Does my story sound familiar? Perhaps you have gone through a similar struggle, or watched someone you love suffer from breathing problems. Let me share with you that life does not have to be this way. If you are plagued by asthma, chronic obstructive pulmonary disease, emphysema, chronic bronchitis, allergies or other breathing issues, what I have learned and now teach will change your life.

Sasha suggested I try the Buteyko Breathing Normalization Method and gave me an earlier edition of this book, which is now in your hands. That's how I first learned about Konstantin Buteyko's discovery and his method. In 1954, Dr. Buteyko discovered that the cause of asthma and breathing difficulties as well as some other diseases was hyperventilation. Since hyperventilation can be lethal, the body does its best to protect itself from it. One of the defense mechanisms is a spasm created in bronchial tubes, which leads to coughing fits and suffocation. Another one is excessive mucus. By doing this, the human body tries to narrow air channels and reduce air consumption. Dr. Buteyko created a breathing method which helps reduce air consumption. As a result, the person stops hyperventilating and his overall health is restored.

As I started learning the concepts of Dr. Buteyko's discovery, I realized that I was indeed, hyperventilating. At first, I followed this book without any supervision or professional advice. The techniques helped somewhat, but I was not improving as much as I needed to. Since this was the only thing that seemed to help me at this point, Sasha and I decided to call the Buteyko Clinica in Moscow and find out if the doctors there could improve my condition. We were fortunate enough to reach Dr. Ludmila Buteyko, the wife and the closest colleague of Konstantin Buteyko. As we were now convinced my asthma was incurable, Sasha tentatively asked Lyudmila Buteyko if there was any chance of improving my condition. "Of course, we can cure his asthma!" she replied. The strength and certainty of her voice came through loud and clear.

We immediately purchased airline tickets and prepared to leave for Moscow. Sasha is Russian, and had previously lived in Moscow, so we were able to stay with her family. I started my treatment in the Clinic right away, with Sasha translating the instructions and advice for me. The Medical Director of the Clinic, Dr. Novozhilov, personally took me through each step of the method, applying and modifying it to the specifics of my condition. With his supervision, I was doing various relaxation and breathing exercises both in the Clinic and at home every evening.

It was amazing how quickly my symptoms vanished. The coughing and constriction was gone, and I no longer needed to be "rescued" by my inhaler or other drugs. Soon after, I was able to stop taking my medication. My fear of dying from suffocation also disappeared. My breathing was fine. My teachers, Ludmila Buteyko and Andrey Novozhilov, saved and changed my life.

My disease was tamed and my body was returning to the good health I had known but lost. I felt like I had a new and better life, as if death had passed me by.

What became the turning point in my life was just another day for the staff of the Clinic. The Clinic was

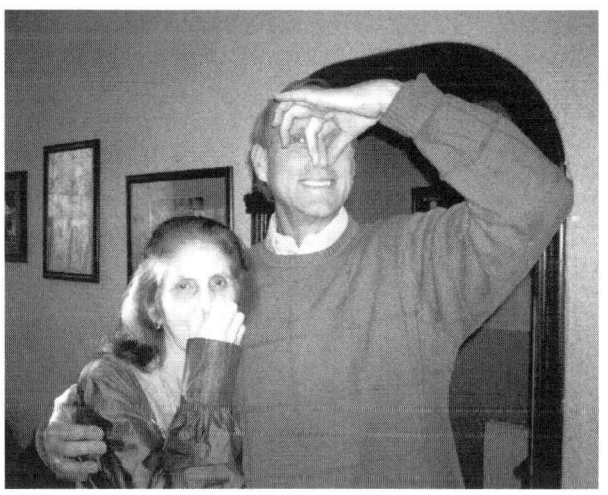

Ludmila Buteyko and Thomas Fredricksen are doing breath holds together.

founded by Konstantin Buteyko twenty-two years ago. Since that time, countless individuals have been cured of asthma and breathing difficulties. The application of the Buteyko Method results in a very significant or total reduction of all symptoms. The method also improves the general sense of well-being, due to its positive effect on the immune and metabolic systems. Thousands of people who suffered from asthma and breathing difficulties are now able to live healthy and productive lives, free of drugs, thanks to the discovery of Dr. Konstantin Buteyko and the Buteyko Method, and to the lifelong dedication to this cure by Ludmila Buteyko and Andrey Novozhilov, MD and their staff in Moscow.

Breathing Center

In 2008, Sasha and I ended up spending an entire month working with the staff of Clinica Buteyko. We realized that if we learned the Buteyko Method thoroughly, we could share this miracle with others who continue to suffer as I had. We both completed an intensive internship at the Clinica and earned the title of Buteyko Method Specialists.

At the end of our training in Moscow, we were asked by Ludmila Buteyko and Andrey Novozhilov, MD to formally and exclusively represent them in the United States. They explained to us that there is a need for an organization that would properly promote the patented Buteyko Method.

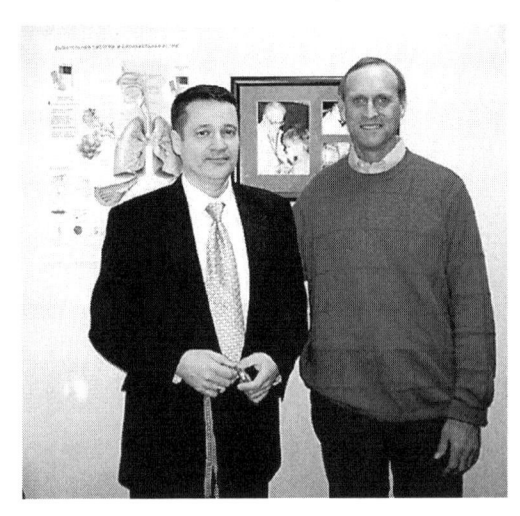

Andrey Novozhilov (left) and Thomas Fredricksen at the Clinica Buteyko. Moscow, 2009

Upon returning to the United States, in conjunction with the Moscow clinic, we formed the Buteyko Center USA, which was later renamed Breathing Center.

Now, the Breathing Center offers educational courses to adults and children who are in need of better health. Additionally, consultations with Dr. Novozhilov, MD, are through our website, www.BreathingCenter.com. The Center also organizes professional trainings for those who wish to teach this method.

Breathe To Heal

Konstantin Buteyko felt that a patient could achieve total success only if he or she worked together with a certified specialist. Nevertheless, Dr. Novozhilov's manual, which is a part of this book, provides an excellent place to start learning the Buteyko Breathing Normalization Method. This expanded volume contains our seventh revision of Dr. Novozhilov's original work, which helped numerous people to tame their breathing difficulties and improve their health.

This volume also presents the historical texts written by Dr. Buteyko. For a first time, this precious work is published in English.

In addition, Sasha Yakovleva added a great deal of information, which will help you to learn about Dr. Buteyko's extraordinary life and his amazing discovery, especially the role it plays to preserve and improve children's health. I also want to mention Sasha's interview with Dr. Packman, the medical consultant of the Breathing Center, who explained in depth the ramifications of hyperventilation, not only for people suffering from asthma but for anyone who over breathes.

We are also pleased to share the stories of some of our students and their experiences with the Breathing Center on their pathway to health.

Study and use this material diligently. Don't stop carrying your inhaler, and don't alter your medication without consulting your medical doctor. You now have an educational process in front of you. If you study and apply it carefully, then you will achieve what thousands of others have in the last several decades: freedom from respiratory problems. "*Breathe To Heal*" as so many of us have done now.

I know from my own experience that the cure is within your grasp. My prayers go out for your excellent health, and I offer you support on your path to perfect health in any way I can. Please don't hesitate to reach out for help and guidance. Breathing Center staff is available the moment you need us. I pray that you will learn and apply the Breathing Normalization method. I promise it will change your life.

By Thomas Fredricksen

SECTION 2: UNDERSTANDING OVER-BREATHING

By Sasha Yakovleva

**Advanced Breathing Normalization Specialist
Co-founder of BreathingCenter.com**

Asthma: The Conventional Treatment Versus The Buteyko Therapy

A conversation between Andrey E. Novozhilov, MD, the Medical Director in Clinica Buteyko Moscow and Sasha Yakovleva, Advanced Breathing Normalization Specialist and co-founder of BreathingCenter.com.

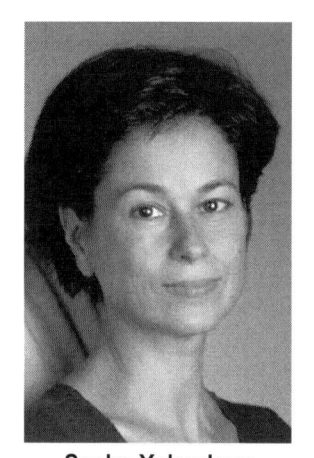

Sasha Yakovleva

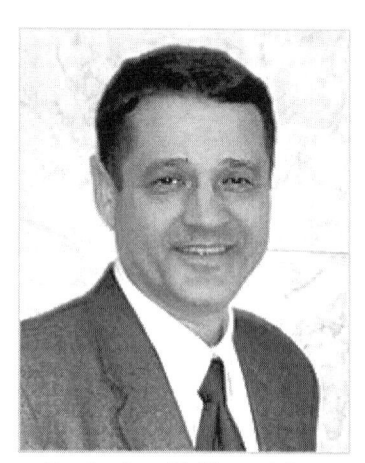

Dr. Andrey E. Novozhilov

Sasha: Asthmatics who have applied the Buteyko Breathing Normalization Method often say, "I cured my asthma!" Nevertheless, from a doctor's perspective, this statement is incorrect. As a medical doctor, could you please explain why conventional medicine considers asthma to be an incurable disease?

Dr. Novozhilov: From the perspective of conventional medicine, asthma is triggered by chronic allergic inflammation of the bronchial tubes. As a result of this, a person with asthma experiences a reversible airflow obstruction, which means that his or her air passages narrow from time to time. This is normally accompanied by bronchospasm, edema and extra mucus, causing asthmatics to struggle with shortness of breath, wheezing, chest tightness, coughing and suffocation attacks.

When this allergic inflammation of the bronchial tubes becomes more active, the airways become narrower, and as a result asthma symptoms become stronger and appear more frequently. When allergic inflammation quiets down to almost nothing, asthmatics forget about their disease as if they never had it.

Unfortunately, allergic inflammation of the bronchial tubes never stops. It lies in ambush, waiting for an opportunity to become active again. Sooner or later this happens, as a result of a person coming in contact with allergens, viruses, pollutants, or even simply cold air. Then the intensity of the inflammation starts increasing again, the air passages become smaller, and consequently, the asthmatic starts experiencing shortness of breath, coughing and other symptoms.

When this happens, doctors normally prescribe steroid-based medications, since no other type of medication is capable of reducing allergic inflammation in the bronchial tubes. So steroids tame the asthma, and an asthmatic is given another chance to forget about his or her disease—until allergic inflammation kicks in again.

Sasha: *So, to stop asthma completely, it is necessary to stop the allergic inflammation of the bronchial tubes. Is it possible to achieve this goal by applying medication?*

Dr. Novozhilov: As of today, there is no medication capable of achieving this goal. Moreover, even a possibility of creating this medication is not feasible since doctors still don't know the main cause of allergic inflammation of the bronchial tubes, and don't fully understand the mechanisms of its development.

Therefore, since doctors have no means of eliminating allergic inflammation, they have to label asthma "an incurable disease." The only thing they can do is to control asthma by reducing or preventing its symptoms with various drugs, including steroids.

Sasha: *Would you explain how the work of K.P. Buteyko, MD-PhD differs from the conventional medical outlook on asthma? What is its theoretical basis?*

Dr. Novozhilov: Doctor Buteyko proved that a deficiency of carbon dioxide (CO_2) in the lungs must be present in order for allergic inflammation of the bronchial tubes to appear or to flare up.

It is not difficult to verify this scientific hypothesis by observing asthmatics who apply the Buteyko Method. When asthmatics start correcting the CO_2 deficiency in their lungs, the allergic inflammation of the bronchial tubes quiets down proportionally, and consequently, the narrowing of the air passages reduces and occurs less frequently. When the concentration of CO_2 becomes stable at the level of the medical norm, allergic inflammation of the lungs disappears completely, and together with it, all asthma symptoms.

Sasha: *Do all asthmatics experience shortage of CO_2 in the lungs? Is their CO_2 level always below the medical norm?*

Dr. Novozhilov: Yes. If a person has been diagnosed with asthma, the level of CO_2 in his or her lungs is always below the norm.

Sasha: *And why is that?*

Dr. Novozhilov: The loss of CO_2 is a result of excessive breathing, which is always present in case of asthma. It is easy to notice that asthmatics are mouth-breathers; their breathing is heavy, often noisy, possibly accompanied by obvious movements of the shoulders, chest or abdominal area. Even visually, this breathing does not look healthy! Doctors call it "hyperventilation of the lungs." Hyperventilation causes asthmatics to lose CO_2, and this is what creates the deficiency.

Doctor Buteyko was the first in the history of health and healing to suggest using a *gradual reduction of breathing* as an asthma treatment. When breathing becomes quiet and gentle, hyperventilation is reduced or eradicated. As a result, the level of CO_2 in the lungs increases, and eventually, becomes normal.

Sasha: *To summarize, Doctor Buteyko's approach helps to reduce allergic inflammation of the bronchial tubes. Can we say that his method produces the same effect as steroids?*

Dr. Novozhilov: By eliminating CO2 shortage in the lungs, the Buteyko Method reduces allergic inflammation of the bronchial tubes, so it does result in the same effect as the intake of steroids. Nevertheless, there is a significant difference: steroids are not capable of ending allergic inflammation, whereas Buteyko Method is. A good example of this is Dr. Buteyko's wife, Ludmila Buteyko. For many years she had been suffering from severe suffocation attacks due to her asthma. She even experienced several clinical deaths. When she met Konstantin Buteyko and learned how to apply his method, her suffocation attacks stopped, and for the next forty years she did not experience any asthma symptoms, even when she caught a very bad cold. This indicates that the allergic inflammation in her bronchial tubes was completely extinguished. This happened because the level of CO2 in her lungs was always equal to the medical norm or even higher. Under these conditions, allergic inflammation of the bronchial tubes is impossible and cannot be provoked.

Sasha: I'd like to mention that there is another very significant difference between Dr. Buteyko's Breathing Normalization and steroids. Dr. Buteyko's method does not have any negative side effects, whereas long-term steroid intake can cause serious health problems.

Dr. Novozhilov: Buteyko Breathing Normalization is a holistic method: its application not only removes asthma symptoms, but also strengthens overall health, improving the efficiency of the human body as a unified system. The effective functioning of the human body, which we commonly call "health," is possible only when the level of CO2 remains normal.

Sasha: Yet, doctors often say, "Are you trying to increase CO2 in an asthmatic? The level of CO2 in his blood is already so high that he can die from it!"

Dr. Novozhilov: Yes, doctors who have not studied the scientific discovery of K.P. Buteyko often make this type of statement.

It is important to understand that when it comes to asthma, the goal of the Buteyko Method is not an abstract increase in the level of CO_2, but the elimination of CO_2 insufficiency specifically in the lungs—NOT in the blood!—since the development of allergic inflammation of the bronchial tubes and the reversible airflow obstruction depend on an under-supply of CO_2 *in the lungs*.

In a healthy person who does not have asthma, the gas exchange between the lungs and the blood is normal, which results in the concentration of CO_2 in the lungs and the blood being approximately the same. If there is a CO_2 shortage in the lungs, then there will be a CO_2 shortage in the blood.

Conversely, if a person suffers from asthma, especially in its severe form, the gas exchange between the lungs and the blood can be impaired. Because of this, the levels of CO_2 in the lungs and the blood can differ. Any asthmatic, whether he or she has a severe, mild, or light form of asthma, has CO_2 deficiency in his or her lungs. However, the concentration of CO_2 in his or her blood can be anywhere in a range from too low to dangerously high.

Sasha: *Let's take a person suffering from a severe form of asthma. He has CO_2 shortage in his lungs and an excess of CO_2 in his blood. Applying the Buteyko therapy, this person reduces his air intake, thus gradually eliminating the shortage of CO_2 in his lungs. What effect would it have on the CO_2 level in his blood? According to what you're saying, it will not increase, but rather reduce? Is this correct?*

Dr. Novozhilov: This is correct. The lungs of a person suffering even from a severe form of asthma are not damaged completely, but only partially. Buteyko breathing reduction will protect his or her lungs from any further damage. In addition, it will make the functioning of the uninjured areas more effective. This will improve the gas exchange process, making it more efficient. As a result, excess CO_2 in the arterial blood will get removed faster, accelerating the improvement of his or her overall health.

Sasha: *Let's go back to the discussion of the goal of Dr. Buteyko's approach: restoring the CO2 level in the lungs to the medical norm. Why is this parameter essential for our health?*

Dr. Novozhilov: CO2 shortage leads to oxygen deficiency in the body. It damages the nervous system and negatively affects the metabolic functions and the immune system. As a result, the body becomes less functional and can expire prematurely.

Sasha: *Why is the body of an asthmatic not capable of maintaining CO2 at the normal level? Is it due to the disease called "asthma"?*

Dr. Novozhilov: No, it is because of chronic hyperventilation. It is important to understand that Dr. Buteyko saw the human body as a self-regulating system. One of its main objectives is to maintain CO2 at the normal level. From this perspective, the key manifestation of asthma—the reversible airflow obstruction—is not a disease, but a compensatory reaction to the loss of CO2 caused by hyperventilation. By narrowing the air passages, the body is trying to force the person to breathe less to prevent a further loss of CO2, which could be dangerous to survival.

Sasha: *It seems that the main disagreement between the conventional medical approach and Dr. Buteyko's approach lies in the interpretation of the meaning of the key manifestation of asthma—the narrowing of the air passages. Conventional medicine believes that this indicates that the asthmatic is not receiving enough air, and therefore, has difficulties breathing. Because of that, traditional doctors often recommend that asthmatics breathe more and deeper. Buteyko-trained doctors read the same bodily message differently. For them, narrowing of the air passages indicates that asthmatics consume too much air, and that their bodies are trying to reduce this excessive air intake. Therefore, Buteyko doctors recommend that asthmatics breathe less and breathe gentler.*

Doctor Novozhilov: The hypothesis of "insufficient air intake" can be checked by measuring the lung ventilation of asthmatics. It is not scarce, but rather, excessive. An asthmatic's lung ventilation exceeds the norm by at least 1.5-2 times, even much more when asthma symptoms become stronger, or during an attack. A healthy person consumes about 6 liters of air per minute, while an asthmatic pushes air through his or her lungs at a rate of 10-40 liters per minute.

Once you recognize that hyperventilation is detrimental to overall health, it becomes clear that the reversible airflow obstruction in asthmatics plays a positive role. It is the body's attempt to maintain homeostasis by forcing a reduction in breathing in order to stop the loss of CO_2.

Sasha: *So, from Doctor Buteyko's perspective, the bronchial tubes narrow in order to force asthmatics to consume less air. By doing this, the body is trying to stop the loss of CO_2 in the lungs, which is dangerous for life. How does the Buteyko asthma treatment affect this process?*

Doctor Novozhilov: By learning how to control and reduce their breathing, asthmatics start normalizing the gas exchange and the level of CO_2 in their lungs. As this normalization progresses, the defense mechanisms against the loss of CO_2—which comprise all the well-known symptoms of asthma—are not needed anymore, and as a result, symptoms disappear. Thus, application of Buteyko Breathing Normalization can lead to complete elimination of asthma, as well as effective prevention of the disease.

Sasha: *Now let's talk about medication. The Buteyko Method is considered drug-free. Based on this, people often assume that Konstantin Buteyko was against any medication.*

Doctor Novozhilov: This assumption is incorrect.

The Buteyko Method helps asthmatics to reduce or eliminate hyperventilation. With application of the method over time, asthmatic symptoms get reduced or eliminated, and as a result, the need for medication to control symptoms is gradually reduced and is eventually eliminated.

Nevertheless, in some cases steroid-based medication does need to be used, but only temporarily. Unlike conventional doctors who normally prescribe high dosages of steroids and long courses of treatment, Dr. Buteyko's steroid treatment protocol allows for a significant reduction in dosage, and shortens the length of time that steroids are needed. This greatly lessens negative side effects and allows asthmatics to eventually become drug-free.

Sasha: *I believe this is very important for any asthmatic! I have met parents of very young children whose doctors have told them that their sons and daughters have to stay on steroids for their whole lives. It's terrifying for me to think how this long-term intake of hormones would affect their health!*

Doctor Novozhilov: To take steroids or not? For how long? And when to stop taking them? These questions are essential for all asthmatics. Answers depend on the intensity of allergic inflammation of the bronchial tubes. Since the traditional medical treatment of asthma cannot stop allergic inflammation, doctors have no choice but to recommend to their patients a periodic and often long-term intake of steroids. This is the only way they can control asthma. But by normalizing the level of CO_2 in the lungs, the Buteyko Method can stop allergic inflammation and eliminate any possibility of its recurrence. The result is that steroids are never needed again.

Speaking about children versus adults, the Buteyko Method normally helps children more quickly and more effectively than adults. Most children are capable of learning how to reduce their breathing during their first visit to our Clinica. Then, within one to two months of regular practice, children usually stop taking steroids because they stop experiencing symptoms.

Sasha: *What do doctors in Clinica Buteyko Moscow think about bronco-dilating medication, such as rescue inhalers? Following Buteyko's rationale, the body of an asthmatic narrows air passages in order to maintain health. But at the same time, traditional doctors often recommend that asthmatics take medications which widen air* *passages. Is this medication conducive to the eradication of asthma and overall improvement in health?*

Doctor Novozhilov: Any medication which increases airflow to the lungs should be used only in emergency situations, such as when a suffocation attack has to be stopped swiftly. The regular use of bronchodilators while a person continues to hyperventilate causes narrowing of the air passages more often and more intensely, which increases production of mucus, coughing and other symptoms. This happens because bronchodilators remove the body's natural defense mechanism against hyperventilation, so the body has to work even harder to compensate.

Sasha: *Perhaps we could say that bronchodilators disarm the asthmatic's body, but the body does not want to give up, and it starts fighting for its own health more aggressively.*

Doctor Novozhilov: We can say so. In order to maintain its homeostasis, the body has to utilize stronger defense mechanisms, which leads to a more severe form of asthma, and possibly even lung damage.

Dr. Buteyko discovered through his research that prior to the widespread use of bronchodilators, asthma was considered a rare and rather mild ailment. By virtue of the periodic narrowing of the air passages, asthmatics were able to maintain adequate levels of CO_2 in their lungs. So at that time people did not die from asthma. In fact, asthmatics were known for having long life spans and not experiencing any health problems besides asthma.

Sasha: *Why is that?*

Doctor Novozhilov: I've already explained that hyperventilation is harmful and can lead to death. To stop this process, the body of the asthmatic activates a variety of compensatory mechanisms. In earlier times, before the advent of bronchodilators, asthmatics were able to maintaining adequate levels of CO_2, and therefore, the normal functions of metabolism and the immune system. So, besides asthma symptoms, they rarely experienced any other health issues.

To understand this, it is important to recognize that asthmatics are not the only ones who experience hyperventilation. But compared to other people, asthmatics possess a unique compensatory mechanism—periodic narrowing of air passages—which prevents the loss of vital CO2 and further deterioration of their health.

Sasha: *What has changed in our modern world?*

Doctor Novozhilov: Well, breathing patterns are greatly determined by lifestyle. Our contemporary lifestyle that is based on comfort, sedentariness, excessive eating, and the use of caffeine, sugar and drug intake supports hyperventilation. Because of that, asthma has become epidemic. Today, asthma is in the process of spreading throughout the world, with a speed which reminds me of the plague epidemics during the Middle Ages.

At the same time, the widespread use of medication which defeats periodic narrowing of the airways has created the situation we have now, in which the deterioration of asthmatics' health has become typical. Consequently, today people often die from asthma.

Sasha: *What is a solution to this situation?*

Doctor Novozhilov: The history of medicine reveals that a disease can be cured only when its cause is known. The plague was eradicated only after the discovery of the pathogen causing it. This discovery made creation of a vaccine feasible, and thus, saved Europe from extinction.

Many scientific and medical laboratories are engaged in an ongoing effort to find an asthma cure. However, conventional medicine continues to state that, "asthma is incurable." What does this tell us? That conventional medicine does not know the cause of asthma. And here I am referring to the main cause of this disease—hyperventilation—the removal of which brings about the cure for an asthmatic and provides prevention. And of course it was all the way back in the 1960s that Soviet doctor and physiologist **Konstantin Buteyko announced that he had discovered the cause of asthma, and offered a treatment to cure it**.

Sasha: *This being the case, why does conventional medicine not accept Doctor Buteyko's discovery? Why is the Buteyko Method such an unusual story when it comes to acceptance of great medical discoveries?*

Doctor Novozhilov: Actually, the history of medical discoveries tells us the opposite: the Buteyko story is very typical! None of the significant discoveries made by doctors, geniuses of their times, were accepted right away by their colleagues. In fact, they were met with distrust and often ridiculed. One example is the brilliant discovery of the Austrian doctor Ignaz P. Semmelweis, who in the 19th century suggested that surgeons disinfect their hands prior to performing surgery. This was a revolutionary idea! At that time, surgeons would often assist a woman in labor right after examining a corpse—without washing their hands!

Today, of course, this would be unimaginable. But back then, this was an unchallengeable medical routine. At that time, women in labor would regularly die from blood poisoning, but doctors were unable to understand the cause, because the existence of microbes was unknown. Even though Semmelweis' implementation of his ideas proved that his recommendations would reduce the death rate of these women by 80%, it was simply not enough for doctors to accept the idea of disinfection. They called Semmelweis' revolutionary discovery quackery. His scientific work was not forgotten only because of the efforts of the relatives of pregnant women who began insisting that doctors wash their hands prior to helping with deliveries. Many years later, when the existence of microbes was proven via observations made through microscopes, conventional medicine finally accepted Semmelweis' discovery and implemented it.

Sasha: *Well, what do you say about that? Let's hope that one day conventional medicine will also accept the revolutionary discovery of Dr. Buteyko!*

Doctor Novozhilov: Every day, more people all over the world are finding out about his discovery. Asthmatics reduce their breathing, and by doing so are able to reduce or even stop their asthma symptoms. The truth cannot be concealed! I have no doubts that sooner or later Dr. Buteyko's Breathing Normalization Method will be accepted by conventional medicine.

Sasha: *Let's hope that it will happen soon, since it would greatly improve health, and even save lives of millions adults and children suffering from asthma!*

Hyperventilation and its Ramifications, Including Asthma

Ira J. Packman MD from Pennsylvania suffered from asthma but was able to improve his condition greatly by taking Breathing Normalization training at the Breathing Center. After thoroughly examining the work of Dr. Buteyko and Dr. Novozhilov, he became a strong advocate of Breathing Normalization. Sasha Yakovleva interviewed Dr. Packman regarding his view of the Buteyko Method, which resulted in the article below.

Dr. Packman: First, I want to say that Dr. Buteyko's concept regarding the origins and causes of many diseases, especially asthma, is radically different from what medical schools teach.

According to all medical schools (whether allopathic, osteopathic or homeopathic), hyperventilation is the result of certain diseases, not the cause. That's why doctors say, "You have chronic anxiety disorder, and therefore, you hyperventilate." Or, "You have chronic pain," or "depression," or "asthma," etcetera, and "therefore, you hyperventilate."

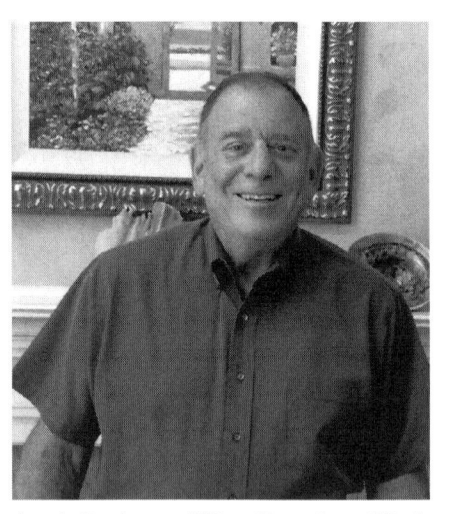

Ira J. Packman MD, a Board certified Internal Medicine Physician, member of American Medical Association

Dr. Buteyko stated, "No, **hyperventilation is not the result of various diseases; it is the cause!**" His concept is revolutionary and may be *too simple* for many academicians to accept.

Sasha: How does over-breathing, or hyperventilation, cause asthma and many other diseases?

Dr. Packman: Since the lungs are a part of the respiratory system, the effect of hyperventilation within the lungs is the easiest to explain and understand. The effects of hyperventilation on the whole body (systems and organs not related to breathing) are more complex.

The systemic ramifications of chronic hyperventilation are numerous. All of them are caused by a low level of CO_2 in the lungs, which causes a decrease in the level of CO_2 in the blood. In the case of asthma, the low level of CO_2 in the lungs causes spasm of the airways. This spasm, which is the cause of wheezing, is the body's attempt to retain the CO_2 in the lungs to correct the problem. Long-term, this shortage of CO_2 in the lungs causes a compensatory response throughout the whole body. Every place where the body produces or excretes CO_2 will attempt to increase the CO_2 level in the body to correct the deficiency caused by chronic hyperventilation.

These reactions throughout the body are the result of the body's ongoing efforts to maintain homeostasis, the condition of balance which is its most comfortable state.

Sasha: *In other words, the body is always trying to stay as healthy as possible, right? Would you please elaborate on how homeostasis works?*

Dr. Packman: All the main functions of the body are controlled by feedback mechanisms. For example, if your blood sugar is too high, the body will respond by creating more insulin to bring the level of sugar down. This is how the body maintains its balance. No matter what the circumstances are, homeostatic mechanisms are in play to bring us back into a physiologic balance. Some of the physiologic parameters controlled in this way include body temperature, glucose levels, hormone levels, mineral balance and others, but most importantly, acid/alkaline balance—pH.

Since pH affects all functions of the body, its control mechanisms are very sensitive and responsive. If pH changes, the body will do anything it can to bring it back to normal.

Hyperventilation and its Ramifications, Including Asthma

Sasha: *Does hyperventilation affect pH?*

Dr. Packman: When people chronically hyperventilate, their pH changes and their pH control system gets activated.

Sasha: *So, what happens to a person who is hyperventilating? Let's say that someone is sitting in a chair and breathing really fast and heavily for a minute or so? What will be the result of it?*

Dr. Packman: The lungs will blow off too much CO_2, lowering the CO_2 level inside the lungs, and therefore lowering the CO_2 level in the blood. As a result, the blood pH will go higher than the norm, becoming more "basic," or alkaline. By the way, normal pH is 7.4; 7.3 is considered Acidotic; 7.5 is Basic or Alkaline.

That is acute hyperventilation. "Acute" means "quickly." In this case, the pH is changing so quickly that the body cannot adjust. As a result, a person will start feeling light-headed, might experience shortness of breath, his or her muscles will cramp, his heart will race, his chest will tighten, he can get tingling or numbness in his fingertips or toes, he might feel chest pressure or pains—ultimately a person can pass out.

Sasha: *But what if a person is breathing just a bit faster and deeper than normal, and does it for several years. It is not noticeable for him or the people around him? Yet his lungs regularly process excessive volumes of air.*

Dr. Packman: This person is also hyperventilating, because he or she is constantly exchanging more air than needed. So, in this case a person also blows off too much CO_2, which changes his pH.

Since this person hyperventilates chronically, the physiologic state of the body is "pathologic" or diseased. In this situation the body starts doing multiple things to correct the pH. Until the underlying cause of the pH abnormality is corrected—hyperventilation—the body cannot return to a healthy state.

Sasha: *When pH changes due to hyperventilation or any other reason, does the body try to correct this situation? Does it make an attempt to bring it closer to the norm?*

Dr. Packman: Of course! The body always struggles to keep its acid/base balance correct. It expends a lot of energy on this because every metabolic and physiologic process in the body is pH-dependent. Whether absorbing nutrients from the bowel or making urine, all the reactions in the body are set up to occur at the pH of 7.4.

So, there are two ways the body can correct pH in the blood. First is a quick way through the lungs. And there is also a slow way, which is through the kidneys.

Sasha: *Would you please explain how the body corrects pH in the blood through the lungs?*

Dr. Packman: When the pH changes, the body quickly responds by changing the breathing. If the pH becomes more acid, the body starts breathing much faster in order to get rid of CO_2 and bring pH back up to the norm.

If pH becomes more alkaline, the body starts breathing slower or starts to wheeze, in an attempt to accumulate CO_2 and bring pH back down to the norm.

Sasha: *And what is the second, the slow way to correct pH through the kidneys? How does this work?*

Dr. Packman: If pH changes, and stays off norm for a long period of time, then the kidneys have to correct this problem in order to prevent other organs and systems from failing.

If a person chronically hyperventilates, he drops the CO_2 level in his blood, and his pH goes up, becoming more alkaline. In this case, the kidneys will excrete more bicarbonate (HCO_3), which is a combination of CO_2 and water—$H_2O + CO_2 = HCO_3$. The kidneys change the pH by changing the amount of bicarbonate in the urine, which directly affects the bicarbonate and CO_2 levels in the blood.

Sasha: *Is the excretion of this bicarbonate damaging for overall health?*

Dr. Packman: Yes. You see, in order to get rid of bicarbonate, the kidneys also have to lose molecules of magnesium, phosphorus, calcium, potassium and sodium. So, these vital minerals leave the body through the urine, when normally the body should keep and use them.

Sasha: *Why would the body get rid of the minerals it needs?*

Dr. Packman: Correcting the pH is its priority. To achieve this goal, the kidneys will sacrifice elements which are less important for the survival of the body in order to maintain a normal pH level.

Sasha: *I assume this makes a person chronically depleted of magnesium, phosphorus, calcium, potassium and sodium. This has to impact the body negatively.*

Dr. Packman: It does. These minerals, particularly magnesium, phosphorus and calcium, are essential for many basic functions of the body—for example, the contraction of muscles and the propagation of nerve impulses. Their deficiency negatively affects how the nerves and muscles work, making a person feel dull and weak.

Sasha: *I know that people who hyperventilate almost always feel weak and fatigued.*

Dr. Packman: Hyperventilation affects our energy level. It happens due to the loss of phosphorus and magnesium from the kidneys. Phosphorus is needed to create ATP, Adenosine triphosphate, which is a molecule that stores energy. A lack of phosphorus and magnesium depletes our energy stores, and prevents the body from producing more energy. This affects every single action; anything that the body needs energy for is not going to work well. This includes the immune system, which will lack energy to create antibodies to fight infections, the liver, the gastrointestinal tract, the kidneys, etc. Muscles and nerves are also affected. When you exercise, your muscles are using up energy. At the same time, energy is created inside the muscles by using ATP. If you don't have much ATP stored, your muscles will fatigue quickly.

Sasha: This tells me that there is no single organ or system in the body which does not get affected by hyperventilation! Based on the information you have given, I can say that a person's quality of life and functionality decreases severely!

Dr. Packman: There is another major factor which makes this situation even worse. Chronic hyperventilation creates chronic oxygen deprivation. What are the results of this? It makes a person feel really lousy! His or her memory will become poor, emotions can be raw and uncontrollable, muscles get fatigued, the heart will not function efficiently, the liver will not be making proteins and glucose as it should, the bone marrow will not respond appropriately to the needs of the immune system—it goes on and on like this.

Sasha: How and why does hyperventilation create a state of oxygen starvation? It would be logical to assume that over-breathing provides us with more oxygen since we take in more air.

Dr. Packman: This is counter-intuitive. You see, our blood contains hemoglobin molecules, which load up on oxygen in the lungs and then carry it through the body, releasing it to the tissues and cells—whether it is the liver, the heart, the bowel, and so forth. This process of releasing oxygen is pH-dependent. Christian Bohr was the Danish physiologist who discovered this relationship between pH on the one hand, and hemoglobin, with its propensity to keep or release oxygen, on the other.

Sasha: So hyperventilation makes blood pH more alkaline. How does it affect the release of oxygen to the tissues and cells?

Dr. Packman: If someone is chronically alkaline—let's say his pH is 7.41 or 7.43 instead of 7.4—the hemoglobin molecules will hold on to the oxygen tighter, and will not release a sufficient volume to the rest of the body. As a result, the whole body will become oxygen starved.

When doctors have a critically ill person in an intensive care unit, they always would rather keep him or her a little more acid than alkaline, because this increases oxygenation of the body. In a slightly acid environment—let's say with pH 7.38 instead of 7.4—the hemoglobin molecule releases oxygen easier to all the organs of the body. This relationship between pH and the hemoglobin molecule's propensity to give up or hold onto oxygen is called the *Bohr Effect*.

So, chronic hyperventilation causes the pH in the blood to be chronically too high, or alkaline. This causes chronic oxygen deprivation, and therefore, everything in the body works less efficiently.

Sasha: *So, hyperventilation starts a domino effect of reactions, which is positive in nature—the attempts of the body to maintain homeostasis—and yet they're injurious for overall health. Is this right?*

Dr. Packman: Yes. If a person chronically hyperventilates, the level of CO_2 in his lungs drops, and this causes the pH in the blood to become abnormally high. To correct this situation, the kidney gets rid of bicarbonate. During this process, the body loses essential elements, which negatively affects everything in the body. On top of it, the body becomes less capable of storing and producing sufficient energy, and also it experiences oxygen starvation. So nothing works well!

Sasha: *That's why Doctor Buteyko stated that hyperventilation was not only a cause of asthma but also about one hundred fifty of the most widespread diseases. He also called asthmatics "fortunate" because he believed that their bodies were capable of preventing this "train wreck" by correcting the situation in the very beginning. What would you say about this?*

Dr. Packman: I agree with this statement. What I described with respect to the kidneys' reaction to hyperventilation is the slow response to hyperventilation. It can take days or week for the kidneys to react. The lungs of an asthmatic react to hyperventilation in seconds.

When an asthmatic hyperventilates, his or her pH goes up, becoming more alkaline. This creates the necessity to acidify the blood quickly. How to achieve this?

The body says, "I know! I should spasm up the airways and hold on longer to the CO2-rich air that is about to be expelled! This will increase the CO2 concentration in the air sacs, increase the CO2 concentration in the blood and thus correct the pH." This is exactly what the bodies of asthmatics do. In other words, wheezing is the body's compensatory mechanism to the alkalosis caused by the state of chronic hyperventilation.

Sasha: So, the body of an asthmatic spasms its airways, and as a result a person experiences difficulties breathing—wheezing, tightness of chest, coughing or suffocation.

Dr. Packman: Correct. The body chooses this discomfort over the more serious trouble hyperventilation can create.

Sasha: What happens if Breathing Normalization is applied?

Dr. Packman: It is as if we say to the body, "All right, you want more CO2? Slow down your breathing and you'll have it, so you don't need to spasm anymore."

When an asthmatic starts breathing slowly and through the nose, he or she decreases the volume of air exchanging in the lungs and stops losing a lot of CO2 through exhalation. This increases the level of CO2 inside his air sacs and in the blood; consequently, the pH goes down and becomes normal. The crisis is over! Airways don't need to spasm anymore and constriction is released. As I've already mentioned, the lungs respond incredibly quickly!

By following the recommendations of the Breathing Normalization Method, asthmatics are able to increase the level of CO2 in their lungs and maintain it at a normal level. When this happens, there is no need for their airways to spasm anymore, and no more wheezing, coughing and suffocation attacks.

Sasha: *I remember that in one of your talks, you compared Konstantin Buteyko with Albert Einstein, stating that Dr. Buteyko's work rewrites the book of medicine in the same way Einstein's work changed physics.*

Doctor Packman: By producing his Theory of Relativity, Einstein said to his fellow physicists, "You are all wrong! This is how it really works!" In response, his work was ignored and Einstein had to work in a mailroom sorting letters. Today, of course, his theory is one of the foundations of modern physics.

Currently, Dr. Buteyko's theory that **hyperventilation is the cause of many diseases** seems far-fetched because it contradicts the generally accepted theories of the medical community. To accept this concept, it requires us, the physicians, to completely change the way we look at the cause of most diseases. Dr. Buteyko's approach is radical. The problem we have is that it works. It is up to us to explain it.

That's exactly what Albert Einstein faced. His Theory of Relativity was real, and therefore, the scientific community had to explain why it worked. This is our challenge as physicians: we have to open our minds and accept the fact that the way we think about the causes of many diseases, including asthma, may not be accurate. This seems simple, and yet it is also extremely complicated, because to start thinking differently is not easy.

Einstein's Theory of Relativity changed the way the world looked at energy, mass and movement. It made physicists think differently about concepts they took for granted. I believe that Dr. Buteyko's theory of hyperventilation as the underlying cause of many disease processes, and the ramifications of that theory, will revolutionize the way modern medicine looks at the causes of most diseases.

I would also like to mention my recent realization of the very interesting connection between Dr. Buteyko's work and the theory and practice of homeopathic medicine. In a homeopathic sense, people who chronically hyperventilate have a deficiency of the essential element CO2. In the case of asthma, wheezing is the body's healing response to correct that deficiency. The kidneys also try to achieve the same goal. Buteyko Breathing Normalization is therefore, a homeopathic treatment for hyperventilation. It gives the body back the CO2, the vital element in which it is deficient.

Sasha: *And when this happens, people who are severely ill often feel as though they were given their life back. It makes sense, since CO2 is considered to be a building block of life. It is a scientific fact that without carbon dioxide life on this planet would be impossible. So we had better acknowledge its importance before it is too late.*

Biography of K.P. Buteyko, MD-PhD

K.P. Buteyko, MD-PhD, is a famous Russian physiologist whose contribution into the field of medicine could be compared to Einstein's role in physics. He created a new health philosophy as well as its practical application, which saved the lives and improved the health conditions of numerous people around the globe. Dr. Buteyko discovered that over-breathing (hyperventilation) is extremely damaging for health and that many health problems could be stopped by the Buteyko Breathing Normalization method. This was the first, but not the only discovery of this legendary doctor.

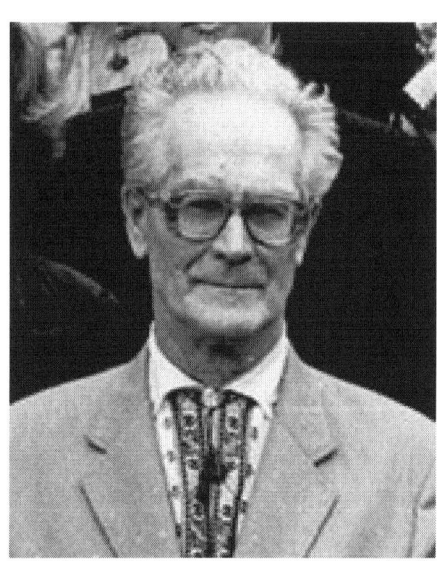

Dr. Buteyko, the originator of the Buteyko Breathing Normalization Method

Konstantin Pavlovich Buteyko was born in 1923 in a small village near Kiev, Ukraine. As a child, he would spend hours quietly observing and examining plants, insects, and almost anything else he encountered. His father was a mechanic, and the boy also liked learning about vehicles. His mother, a schoolteacher, was known to say, "I gave birth to an odd boy," referring to her son's avid curiosity about understanding how things work.

Buteyko saw any mechanism as an intriguing collection of parts, and would be tempted to take them apart. Growing older, he became fascinated by the idea that it is not only the parts that make things work smoothly, but the interaction between them—the balance of a system as a whole, supported by certain constants. This natural progression led him to the Polytechnic College in Kiev, where he began studying engineering.

During his sophomore year, in 1941, German fascists attacked the Soviet Union. Buteyko enlisted and volunteered to go to the frontlines. He spent the next four years in the war zone working as a driver, mechanic, and helper in a medical aid party. He saw many vehicles damaged in battle and was able to fix them. He also saw many human casualties and was frustrated that he did not have the skills to save people's lives. At that time, he viewed the human body as the most superior of all machines, and finding ways to help it operate in the most effective way became his new goal. He decided to study medicine.

After the war, Buteyko enrolled at First Medical Institute in Moscow, Russia. He was an outstanding student, and soon became known as the handsome young veteran with a sharp intellect and abundant energy—and for having the highest grades. He spent most of his time studying at the library or conducting clinical work. Upon graduating with distinction, he was invited to join the staff at one of Moscow's most elite hospitals. His scientific and clinical supervisors, as well as his friends, were convinced that a bright future was beginning to unfold for this talented doctor.

While still in medical school, Buteyko had specialized in the study of hypertension (also called high blood pressure). Ironically, Buteyko himself developed a malignant form of this; in this case, it was a lethal disease. The hospital whose staff he had joined prescribed him the best medicine available for the treatment of this illness, but his condition only worsened. In the fall of 1952, his health had deteriorated to such a degree that it seemed unlikely he would live for more than a couple of months.

Buteyko was a man of great strength and fortitude who, despite tremendous pain, continued working. One evening, during his night shift at the hospital, he was alone in a room, standing in front of a window and looking up at a star-filled sky. His mind was racing with questions: "What is the cause of my disease? Why do people become ill?" Suddenly, a blinding light flashed outside, and he lowered his gaze to shield his eyes. Looking downward to regain his vision, he suddenly noticed that his chest and belly were moving a great deal as he was breathing. It was common medical knowledge that heavy breathing was a symptom of hypertension, but at this moment, Konstantin had an idea, which later he described as strange: "Could it be," he thought, "that my heavy breathing was not the result of my disease but the cause of it?"

Ever the indefatigable scientist, he immediately began experimenting on himself. First, he decreased his breathing by making an effort to breathe gentler. Within a few minutes, his headache, and the strong pain in his chest and kidneys that had always accompanied him began to subside. Second, he increased his breathing by switching to heavy mouth breathing. His pain came back almost immediately. This was a pivotal moment for Buteyko, one that would change the course of his life.

Many years later, he stated that within these first minutes of discovery, the whole chain of cause and effect appeared before his eyes. He thought, "Over-breathing eliminates CO_2 from the body and consequently creates contractions of bronchi, blood vessels, intestines, and so on. These spasms reduce oxygen delivery to the body, causing oxygen starvation. This increases respiration even more, creating a vicious circle." It immediately became clear to him that many diseases associated with the contraction of blood vessels, such as high blood pressure, coronary artery disease, heart attack, stroke, ulcer, chronic nephritis, and others have a single cause: over-breathing. His thought process continued. "Then, hyperventilation changes pH—the acid-base balance—and causes a disturbance of metabolism. Dysfunctional metabolism transmits immune reactions into allergic, which tells us that allergy could also be caused by hyperventilation, as well as high cholesterol, obesity, or thinness. It also weakens immunity, and thus, people catch colds and other, more serious diseases. The metabolic disorder can become so severe that a tumor will develop. This means that even cancer could be caused by deep breathing."

That night he went to the pulmonological department of the hospital where an asthmatic, fighting suffocation, was trying to gasp as much air as possible.

"Slow down your breathing and breathe less!" Buteyko suggested.

"...but doctor, you've always told me, 'Take a deep breath!'"

"I know; I was wrong. Please breathe gentler," Buteyko insisted.

After a few minutes of slowed breathing, the patient was able to breathe better, and his face regained some color. The asthma attack receded. Both men were surprised by how quickly it was defeated.

Of course, Buteyko was excited by his finding and wanted to enlighten the whole world about it. He knew how tremendously beneficial it would be for people! The next morning, he went to his clinical and academic supervisor and revealed his remarkable discovery. The physician listened carefully, but his reply was not what Buteyko expected. "Don't tell anyone," the doctor insisted, "or you will end up in a mental institution." Stalin was still holding power in Russia and had recently sent many doctors to the Gulag on forged grounds for arrest. His supervisor truly cared about this talented doctor and wanted to protect Buteyko's life. He immediately recognized that his groundbreaking discovery would question the very basis of traditional medicine and make many officials merciless.

But the young doctor was not the type to give up easily. First, he tried his new approach himself. Breathing reduction eliminated his malignant hypertension, and he fully regained his health. Then, he proceeded to test his method on his patients at the hospital. He discovered the result was consistently positive. When his patients increased their breathing, their symptoms worsened. When they reduced their breathing, their symptoms receded and their health improved. By modifying the breathing patterns of his patients, Buteyko was able to achieve much greater results than when he treated them with traditional medication. Additionally, his method did not have any negative side effects. And yet, he could not reveal the results of his work.

It was during this time of personal trial that Dr. Buteyko compared the path of his discovery to that of the Austrian physician Ignaz Semmelweis. In 1847, Semmelweis discovered that sepsis occurring during childbirth in hospitals could be radically reduced by washing hands. At the time, doctors would often switch between dissecting corpses and assisting women in labor without washing their hands. The mortality rate of infants and mothers was incredibly high. Dr. Semmelweis believed that it was possible to reduce it by simply requiring doctors to wash their hands with bleach and lime prior to surgery in order to get rid of microbes, then an unknown concept. Sepsis was attributed to many causes, and Semmelweis's hypothesis, that there was one cause for this fierce blood infection, seemed too simplistic. It was discredited and ridiculed by his peers, and Semmelweis was ostracized by the medical community. After years of fighting for his discovery, he was confined to a mental asylum. Fifty years later, however, Louis Pasteur confirmed Semmelweis's theory by developing the germ theory: "I saw microbes," he said, "but Semmelweis was the one who discovered them."

Similar to Semmelweis, Dr. Buteyko came to the conclusion that many health issues, which are considered by the medical community to be unique diseases, are various symptoms of one disease: over-breathing. Hyperventilation leads to the development of asthma, hypertension, and cancer—many of the world's most common diseases. Buteyko realized that these diseases can be cured by reducing one's breathing, but the idea was just too simple for other medical officials to accept. Facing ridicule and potential incarceration for revealing his discovery, Buteyko had to keep most of his findings secret in order to continue developing his method. The only way his work could possibly gain credibility was if he could collect substantial scientific data to support his theory.

At this time, in the 1960s, a new Academy of Science was developing in the largest city in Siberia. It was a difficult choice, but Dr. Buteyko decided to leave an elite hospital in the most culturally sophisticated city in Russia and move to Siberia, thousands of miles away from the launch of his potentially brilliant career. He saw no other way to collect and assemble the data necessary to raise awareness for his revolutionary discovery. He moved to Akadem-gorodock (literal translation: "the town of academics") where he was offered a job as the head of a scientific and clinical laboratory with abundant funding.

To help in his experiments, Buteyko purchased the best possible medical equipment in the Soviet Union and abroad and also invented his own instruments. One of them was a unique device called the "medical combine," which was capable of simultaneously measuring many bodily functions. The data provided by this equipment confirmed his hypothesis: the level of carbon dioxide in the lungs is the main regulator of many bodily functions, and because of hyperventilation, this level becomes insufficient, therefore offsetting constants of the body and creating various dysfunctions.

Dr. Buteyko and his colleagues also conducted a great deal of clinical work treating seriously ill patients, especially asthmatics. Often, people would be carried into his laboratory and then miraculously walk out of it on their own. Buteyko's reputation grew exponentially. People who were severely ill traveled great distances to be treated by him, and he was besieged with hundreds of letters every day requesting his help. Articles reporting on Dr. Buteyko's successes appeared in the national press, and he became known far and wide for his method.

Buteyko's accomplishments generated envy among his colleagues. One of his medical peers was putting all of his efforts into the development of a new drug to ease asthma symptoms. And here was Konstantin Buteyko offering a natural cure for asthma! Where would the work of this doctor be if Buteyko's method would become officially accepted? Buteyko's main supervisor was a renowned surgeon whose approach to asthma had been to remove the afflicted lung, treat it, and then put it back into the body. Although the effectiveness of this technique was insignificant, he had hoped this work would eventually earn him a Nobel Prize. Dr. Buteyko's discovery and its simplicity was a threat for these and many other medical professionals.

This surgeon gathered a group of doctors and began a campaign to sabotage Dr. Buteyko's work. In 1968, while Konstantin was away on a business trip, a person with an axe broke into his laboratory and chopped up his unique equipment. His staff was dismissed and his data was compromised. Eyewitnesses said that when Buteyko entered the room that was once his sophisticated laboratory, his dark hair started to turn grey. On top of all this, Buteyko received multiple death threats intimidating him into stopping his work. He was once poisoned, and an automobile crash was arranged to kill him. He miraculously survived all of these attempts.

Despite these setbacks, Buteyko was able to continue his work. He had helped a few influential officials who had begged him to cure their "incurable diseases," and after their recovery, they felt obligated to protect him. At some point, Buteyko was offered an opportunity to practice his method in space medicine. At first, it seemed like a beneficial way to advance his work and assure him financial security. But soon it became apparent that this job would drastically limit his ability to help people. This was during the Cold War; agreeing to work with astronauts meant automatically swearing to secrecy. He refused this offer in order to have the freedom to help those in need of his method, rather than have it sequestered for an elite few.

Buteyko was known for his altruism. Sometimes, when his patients were lacking money for transportation or accommodation, Buteyko shared his own very modest resources. After his laboratory was destroyed, he started seeing patients at their homes or in his apartment. At that time, private practice was not legal in the Soviet Union, but Buteyko continued helping people privately on a donation basis. For almost twenty years, Dr. Buteyko was officially unemployed and his name was on the medical black list.

The '80s brought some relief for Buteyko. In 1981, the second official trial of his method took place at the Moscow Medical Academy, in the department for asthmatic children. The results were extremely positive: between 94 and 96 percent were healed. In 1983, twenty-one years after his application, he received a patent with a "top secret" classification for his discovery and the treatment method. In 1985, the Ministry of Public Health of Russia issued instructions and recommendations to all medical professionals to treat patients with his breathing method; however, those instructions were never implemented. In 1987, at the very beginning of the Perestroika (transformation of socialism to capitalism), Dr. Buteyko was finally allowed to establish his own clinic in Moscow. Later, it became known as Clinica Buteyko.

Buteyko Clinic in Moscow was founded by K.P. Buteyko, MD-PhD and his closest and the most devoted colleagues—his wife L.D. Buteyko and her son A.E. Novozhilov, MD; both eventually became co-authors of the Buteyko Method due to their invaluable contribution to the development of the Buteyko Method.

Many people suffering from asthma, allergies, hypertension, kidney problems, cardiological and gastrological issues, immune deficiency, cancer, and other serious diseases were healed at Clinica Buteyko.

Dr. Buteyko also started working with people who were exposed to radiation during the Chernobyl nuclear disaster. An official trial of this work took place in 1990 in Kiev, Ukraine, at the National Scientific Center of Radiation Medicine. The result: 82 percent of patients experienced significant improvements in their health. In 1991, there were two more official trials of the Buteyko Method™. Buteyko's team worked with AIDS patients at the Institute of Epidemiology (Kiev). This study demonstrated positive results with no negative side effects. Later, the same Institute conducted another trial with hepatitis and liver hepatocirrhosis patients. Dr. Buteyko's Breathing Normalization proved to be very effective and was officially recommended for use on patients with such problems.

As many famous doctors and scientists have done, Konstantin used his own body to experiment with his method. He practiced what he referred to as "air fasting" and followed a lifestyle that promoted reduced breathing. His own experience, which his advanced students confirmed, showed that Breathing Normalization leads not only to an improvement of physical health but also to clarity of mind, inner peace, and calmness. Buteyko started his career as a traditional doctor, but by the final period of his life, he developed characteristics of a highly developed spiritual practitioner. He was known to have some clairvoyant abilities, was able to operate on very little sleep or food, and was capable of holding his breath for several minutes. Often, the first question he would ask his patients was, "Do you believe in God?" His methods led him to a point when he did not have any doubts about the leading role of the divine, especially when it comes to healing.

Buteyko understood that the door to personal evolution could be opened through breathing. This is not a new thought; it is a paradigm that was practiced in many ancient cultures. For example, one of the goals of Pranayama, a type of Indian yoga, is to breathe less. A basic meditation in Tibetan Buddhism, which is called Shine (Peace), provides a step-by-step training for developing gentle, reduced breathing. Japanese Samurai would put a feather under their nose and breathe on it. If the feather moved, the trainee would be dismissed from the Samurai army. Russian Orthodox Saints recommended their disciples reduce their breath during prayer, as they believed this would bring them closer to God. Dr. Buteyko's achievement rediscovered the benefits of breath reduction. He had developed a unique health improvement method suitable for modern people—one that was especially valuable for those who are ill.

In 2003, the average lifespan for men in Russia was between 50 and 60 years. Buteyko was 80 years old and active despite the damage caused by the several attempts on his life, including one in 1998, when he was the victim of a street assault. One winter night in Siberia, while walking home, the elderly doctor was brutally attacked by three men who beat him with heavy metal bars. When they thought he was dead, they threw his body into the snow. When he was found, doctors were astonished that he was alive; however, they said his chance of surviving was very slim. He lived and worked for another four years, though his health was greatly damaged.

During this time, he traveled a great deal. His method had gradually begun to be recognized not only in Russia, but also in other countries. He was invited to England to treat Prince Charles, who was suffering from allergies. Buteyko and his wife Ludmila successfully treated the Prince's problem. They also visited Germany, New Zealand, and other countries, informing people about his discoveries and sharing the basic elements of his method.

The day before Buteyko passed away, he asked Ludmila Buteyko to take him to a hospital. She was surprised, given that he was feeling well, but she followed her husband's request. The doctors examined him and concluded that there was nothing wrong. In fact, they happily announced to Ludmila that she should expect her husband to live another 10 or 20 years.

However, he passed away the next day. Why? Ludmila's answer was this: "By that time, he did everything he could to offer the people of this planet the valuable knowledge that could save the lives of many as well as the life of the whole civilization. Unfortunately, his offer was not fully accepted due to a reluctance to change, to go beyond the comfort of stereotypical thinking. He respected this choice; however, felt that his mission on Earth was complete." On May 2, 2003, Konstantin looked at Ludmila, his partner and kindred spirit, smiled, then turned to his right side and effortlessly left his body. It was an auspicious day in Orthodox Christianity, the religion permeating Russian culture—the day when the doors to heaven are opened to all passing away from this world.

Dr. Buteyko passed away but Buteyko Breathing Normalization is alive and better than ever. Today it is offered in Russia by Clinica Buteyko; in the USA, it is exclusively offered by the BreathingCenter.com, which officially represents Clinica Buteyko and the patented Buteyko Method.

By Sasha Yakovleva

Special Thanks to David Wiebe, Susan Lipkins and Tusha Yakovleva

About A. E. Novozhilov, MD

Dr. Buteyko called Dr. Novozhilov "Co-Author" of the Buteyko Method. Both of them established Buteyko Clinica in Moscow. Andrey Novozhilov created main medical programs for treating specific diseases. After Konstantin and Ludmila Buteyko passed away, Dr. Novozhilov became a solo holder of all intellectual property associated with the Buteyko Method.

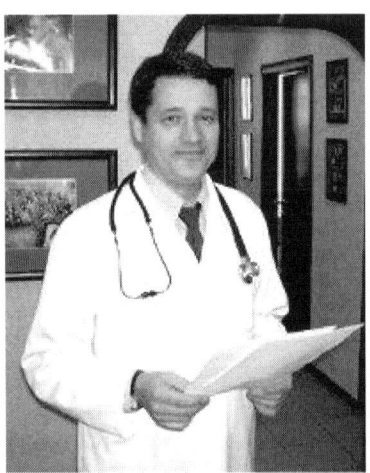

Dr. Andrey Novozhilov

As a nine-year-old boy, Andrey witnessed the clinical death of his mother, Ludmila, two times. She suffered from vicious asthma attacks and cancer, and doctors did not believe Ludmila could survive her disease. Andrey remembers this period as a hopeless time, during which he would often knock on all the doors in their apartment building, asking neighbors to help his mother. People felt sorry for the little boy, but no one was able to help.

One day in 1969, Andrey and Ludmila found a newspaper article about Professor Buteyko. Out of desperation, they wrote him a letter. At that time, Buteyko resided in Siberia, where he worked as the head of a scientific laboratory. Despite his remote location, he was receiving over 200 letters a day from people like Ludmila.

Even though it was impossible to help everyone, Buteyko made his best effort to help as many people as he could. During his next trip to Moscow, he visited Ludmila at home. He attempted to teach Ludmila, but her severe health condition made it impossible for her to comprehend the method. The Professor then decided to teach his method to Andrey, in hopes that he could explain it to his mother. When Dr. Buteyko left, Andrey, gently and patiently, began teaching the method to Ludmila, encouraging her to reduce her breathing. In two weeks, her health improved dramatically, and she was able to return to her normal life. So at the age of nine, Andrey had his first medical experience—saving the life of his own mother.

Later on, Ludmila became the wife of Konstantin Buteyko, which gave Andrey a unique chance to study the Buteyko Method first-hand.

Being greatly impacted by Buteyko's work, Andrey completed his studies and graduated from the First Moscow Medical Institute in 1989. He started working as a general practitioner. He often spent evenings and even nights discussing physiology with Konstantin. He was the one to whom Konstantin passed his medical knowledge.

Dr. Novozhilov is currently the Medical Director of the Buteyko Clinic. In Moscow he sees patients on a daily basis. It is impossible to say how many lives he has saved, or how many people regained their health due to his work. In his approach, Andrey never limits himself to a solely physiological perspective, even though he is an expert in this field. He sees a clear connection between body, mind, and spirit, and believes that every health problem has a reason, which often lies beyond the medical.

SECTION 3:
THE MEDICINE OF THE FUTURE

By Konstantin P. Buteyko, MD-PhD

The renowned physiologist, creator of the Buteyko Method, co-founder of Clinica Buteyko in Moscow

About Asthma

Following is a very important historical document written by Doctor Buteyko. In a very concise way, he explains the cause of asthma and the reason that it often turns into a more dangerous (in fact sometimes even lethal) widespread disease.

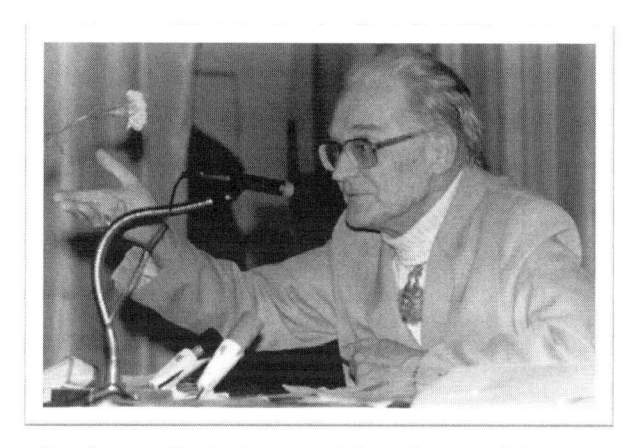

Professor Buteyko, teaching doctors his new asthma treatment

Two hundred years ago asthma was considered a mild ailment. Having asthma generally meant having a long life free of other diseases. But nobody could explain how asthma prevented other diseases or why asthmatics lived longer than other people.

Today we know that asthma is no ordinary disease. Bronchospasm, the main component of asthma, acts as a protective mechanism, maintaining biological constants and important functions to near normal.

And we know, too, that there can be no asthma and no bronchospasm unless the carbon dioxide level in the lungs is abnormally low. Since the metabolism and immune system can only function correctly if the carbon dioxide level is normal, the limit to the asthmatic's carbon dioxide loss protects them for a long and healthy life.

It is this powerful defense mechanism that provides the asthmatic with an improved biological system. Evidently, bronchospasm is one way the organism has been able to adapt to its environment.

Modern drug treatment for asthma is aimed at neutralizing this protective mechanism. The organism then fights back again and again with more intensive bronchospasm, leading to a rapid deterioration of the asthma from drug treatment.

It is not possible to cure asthma by removing a protective mechanism like bronchospasm. Only when the condition responsible for the bronchospasm is removed can asthma be reversed.

The Theory of My Method

Here is another important historical document, published in a printed form for the first time here Dr. Buteyko explains why hyperventilation can trigger not only asthma but many other diseases, including cancer.

Thirty-eight years ago, I announced that a great number of widespread diseases triggered by the lifestyle of our civilization (i.e., bronchial and vasomotor spasms, allergic reactions, etc.) have a common cause: hyperventilation (excessive breathing). I realized that decreasing and thus normalizing the air intake can lead to an individual's recovery. Scientific studies, as well as the basic laws of physiology, biochemistry, and biology, have confirmed this hypothesis. Here are the general postulates of my theory:

When an excessive amount of air is consumed, a large amount of carbon dioxide is removed from the organism, consequently reducing the CO_2 content of the lungs, blood, and tissue cells. A hyperventilation-caused CO_2 deficiency produces pH alkaline shifts in the blood and tissue cells. The pH shifts interfere with all protein (about 1000 in all) and vitamin (about 20) activity, altering the metabolic processes. Therefore, when the pH level reaches the value of 8, the metabolic disorders can cause death.

A CO_2 deficiency also causes spasms in the smooth muscles of the bronchi, cerebral and circulatory vessels, intestines, biliary ducts, and other organs. In the late 19th century, Bronislav Verigo, a Russian scientist from Perm, discovered a peculiar relationship: when CO_2 diminishes from the blood, oxygen binds with hemoglobin and impairs the transport of oxygen to the brain, heart, kidneys, and other organs. In other words, the deeper the breathing, the less oxygen reaches vital organs in the body. This statement forms the basis of my discovery, one that has gone underappreciated until now. This dependency, presented by Verigo, was suppressed and ignored. At the same time, Christian Bohr, a Swedish scientist, made a similar discovery. Later on, this became known as the Bohr Effect.

Hypoxia (oxygen deficiency) in the brain caused by deep breathing triggers intense bronchial and cardiac spasms. Hypoxia in vital organs is counter-balanced by the rise in arterial tension (artery hypertension), which enhances blood circulation and provides the organs with blood. Oxygen starvation, when combined with hyperventilation, causes a false feeling of air deficiency, excites the respiratory center, intensifies breathing, and contributes to the progression of disease.

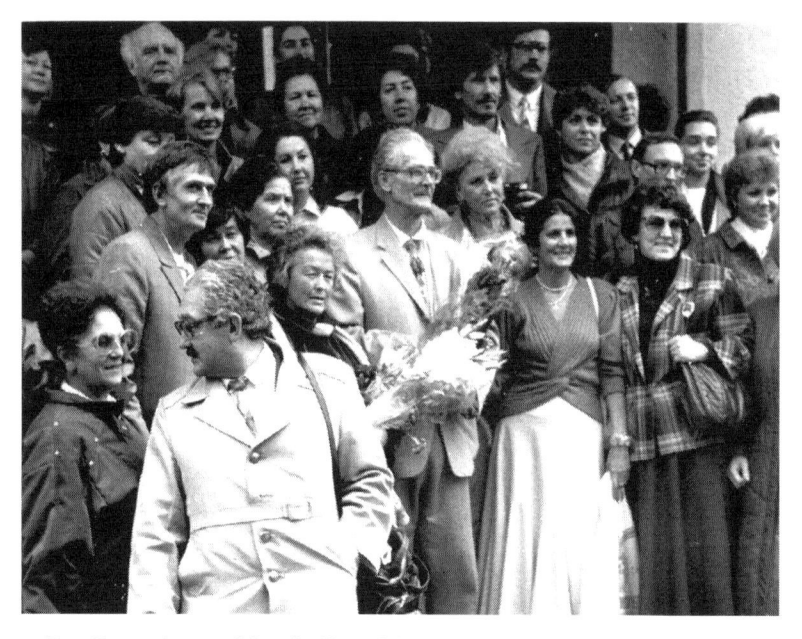

Dr. Buteyko and Ludmila with a group of doctors learning about breathing reduction

A CO2 deficiency in the nerve cells excites all of the structures in the nervous system, thus making the process of breathing even more intense. As a result, oxygen starvation in nerve cells, in combination with metabolic malfunctions and an over-excited nervous system, brings about mental disorders, destroys the nervous system (sclerosis of cerebral vessels), and finally, causes a deterioration of an individual's physical and mental health.

Disorders brought about by hyperventilation are aggravated by factors such as environmental pollution, pesticides, and other chemicals that are found in nutritional products. If we assume this, then the basic principles of Western medicine—the remedial and preventative measures that commonly use over-breathing methods—just add to the development of diseases. Strenuous exercise and drugs, which relax the bronchi and blood vessels (thus increasing the removal of CO_2 from the body), do not improve a patient's condition, but only worsen it.

This is precisely why diseases triggered by the modern environment go untreated and are so widespread. The discovery of the fact that the main cause of such diseases is hyperventilation proves (through experiments) the fallacy of the existing remedial methods and principles.

A hyperventilation test serves as decisive evidence that this method is effective. For example, a patient is offered to increase his breathing and evaluate the result of the well-known command, "Take a deep breath." Within a few seconds or minutes, this deep breathing test will trigger or increase pathological symptoms. Meanwhile, a reduction of the volume of respiration will remove the symptoms almost at the same rate. Thus, the only effective principle for prevention and treatment is to reduce the volume of breathing, thus allowing normal respiratory function to be restored.

This is the basis for the development of mindful control of hyperventilation. The essence of the technique is for a patient, through willfulness and diligence, to lessen his depth of breathing by relaxing the respiratory muscles until he feels a slight air deficit.

Adults and children over three years old can use this method. The method can also be used in obstetrics for expecting mothers and their newborns to teach children healthy physiological principles.

This theory is also directly applicable to space medicine, surgery (preparation for surgical intervention), pedagogy, training of singers and athletes, and more. Medicine, just like other branches of science, requires a comprehensive restructuring. The author considers his ideas, along with other progressive approaches, which have been ignored, as a foundation for the medicine of the future. The top priority is to provide people with information about this method in order to stop the propaganda of deep breathing (over-breathing) in the mass media and to remove over-breathing exercises from health care. The method developed by the author will succeed when every human being realizes that his inborn greed (which applies to breathing) is the cause of diseases and disasters.

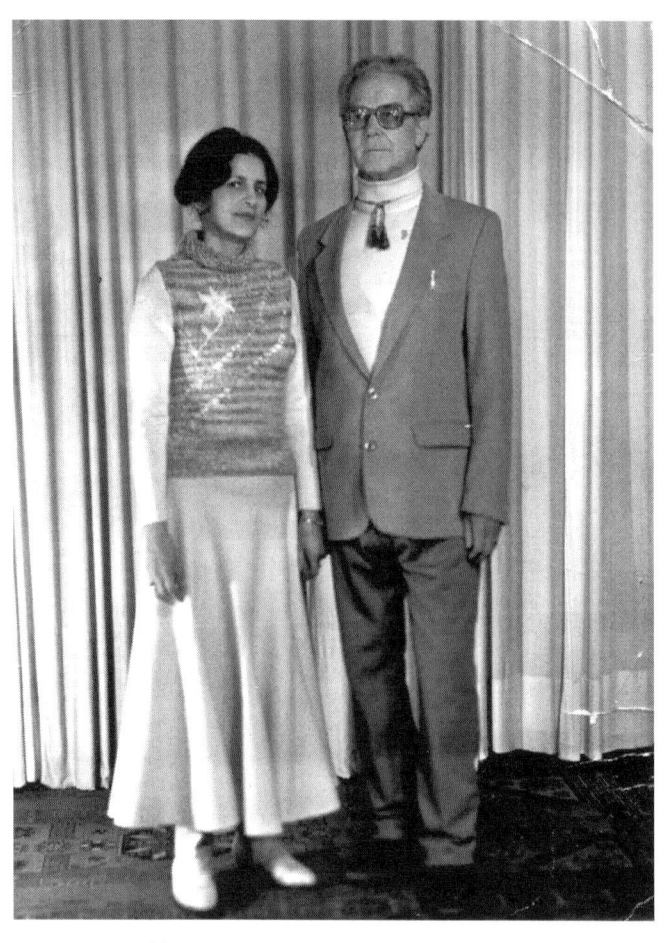

Konstantin and Ludmila Buteyko

List of Health Problems Triggered by Hyperventilation

Dr. Buteyko would often say, "I made a serious mistake when I agreed with my students to present my method as asthma cure, when in fact it can tame not only asthma but many other diseases." Here for a first time, we are presenting the list of All Diseases Reversible by Breathing Reduction as Dr. Buteyko called it. This text, written by K.P. Buteyko MD-PhD, was slightly edited by Ira J. Packman MD to make it easier to understand for people in present times.

1. All Kind of Allergies:
    a. Respiratory allergies
    b. Polyvalent allergy, including pollen disease
    c. Laryngospasm (voice loss)
    d. Allergic conjunctivitis
    e. Food allergies
    f. Drug allergies
    g. False [spasmodic] croup
    h. Pharyngitis
    i. Laryngitis
    j. Tracheitis
2. Asthmatic bronchitis
3. Asthma
4. Chronic Obstructive Pulmonary Disease (COPD)
5. Rhinitis (Chronic cold)
6. Vasomotor rhinitis
7. Frontal sinusitis
8. Maxillary sinusitis
9. Sinusitis
10. Enlarged Adenoids
11. Polyps (polyposis)
12. Chronic rhinosinusitis
13. Pollinosis (hay fever)

14. Angioedema
15. Hives (urticaria)
16. Eczema, including:
    a. Neurodermatitis
    b. Psoriasis
    c. Infant rash
    d. Vitiligo
    e. Ichthyosis
    f. Acne
17. Raynaud's disease (vascular spasms of the upper limbs)
18. Arterial Occlusive Disease
19. Varicose veins
20. Thrombophlebitis
21. Hemorrhoids
22. Hypotension
23. Hypertension
24. Vegetative-vascular dystonia (VVD) or Neurocirculatory Dystonic Disease
25. Congenital heart disease
26. Rheumatoid arthritis (RA)
27. Rheumatic heart disease
28. Diencephalic syndrome
29. Coronary heart disease (CHD), Ischemic heart disease (IHD)
30. Chronic Ischemic heart disease
    a. Rest and exertional angina (pectoris)
    b. Post-infarction cardiosclerosis
31. Heart Rhythm Disorders
    a. Tachycardia
    b. Arrhythmia
    c. Paroxysmal tachycardia (PSVT)
    d. Atrial fibrillation
32. Atherosclerosis
33. Arachnoiditis (post-traumatic, influenzal, etc.)

34. Post-stroke conditions:
    a. Paralysis
    b. Paresis
35. Parkinson's disease (early stage)
36. Hypothyroidism
37. Hyperthyroidism
38. Graves' disease
39. Diabetes
40. Menstruation Disorders
41. Morning sickness
42. Menopausal Disorders
43. Cervical erosion
44. Fibromyoma
45. Fibrocystic Breast Disease (FBD)
46. Infertility
47. Impotence
48. Threatened miscarriage
49. Radicular pain
50. Osteochondrosis
51. Metabolic polyarthropathy
52. Rheumatoid polyarthropathy
53. Dupuytren's contracture (contracture of the palmar fascia)
54. Gout
55. Pyelonephritis
56. Glomerulonephritis
57. Nocturnal urinary incontinence (bed-wetting)
58. Cystitis (urinary bladder inflammation)
59. Kidney stone disease
60. Obesity (all degrees)
61. Lipomatosis
62. Chronic gastritis
63. Chronic cholecystitis
64. Biliary dyskinesia

65. Chronic pancreatitis
66. Gallstone disease
67. Duodenal ulcer
68. Irritable bowel syndrome
69. Peptic ulcers (PUD)
70. Multiple sclerosis
71. Epileptic syndrome, (epilepsy)-convulsive syndrome
72. Schizophrenia (early stage)
73. Connective tissue diseases (cleroderma, systemic lupus erythematosis, dermatomyositis
74. Glaucoma
75. Cataracts
76. Strabismus
77. Farsightedness
78. Radiation sickness
79. Radiation sickness
80. Acute and chronic hepatitis

SECTION 4: BUTEYKO BREATHING MANUAL

By Andrey Novozhilov, MD

Medical Director of Clinica Buteyko in Moscow and its co-founder

Illustrations by
Victor Lunn-Rockliffe

Part 1: Buteyko Theory

Introduction
The Buteyko Method, which includes the Buteyko breathing exercises, is a therapy that enables any form of asthma to be controlled and ultimately cured without medication or with a greatly reduced drug regime.

K.P. Buteyko MD-PhD discovered that hyperventilation is the root cause of asthma. He was the first scientist to attribute constriction of the bronchioles to excessive breathing or hyperventilation. He understood that if hyperventilation could be reversed, asthma symptoms would be controlled. This led to his development of a new therapy aimed at reversing hyperventilation.

The Buteyko Method can reverse all forms of asthma, of any severity, since all forms of asthma result from hyperventilation, which we consider reversible. However, in moderate to severe asthma, it is sometimes necessary to use medication during the recovery process. Medication is always gradually reduced and eventually eliminated with the Buteyko Method. If this occurs, chronic hyperventilation and steroid abuse sometimes results in such severe damage to the adrenal glands that they may not recover completely. In this event, small amounts of steroid supplements will be required permanently.

The Buteyko Method depends on complete patient compliance. Full recovery is only achieved if the patient practices the method diligently. This is commonly not the case. Successful application of the method occasionally also requires changes to unhealthy lifestyle habits. The Buteyko Method is no miracle cure and does not involve any "magic." It is a carefully conceived program aimed at restoring good health.

The method incorporates a simple and effective system for measuring your state of health. This system is based on the breathing measurements such as Positive Maximum Pause (PMP), which is the length of time you can hold your breath with slight discomfort, and Control Pause (CP), which is the length of time you can hold your breath without discomfort (both pauses are described more fully later).

Regular measurement of your breathing provides an objective measure of progress towards normalizing respiratory functions and restoring health.

Today, 60 to 80 percent of asthmatics have a mild form of asthma. In mild asthma, small exacerbations, without a full scale asthma attack, occur no more than twice a week during the day and no more than once a month at night. This level of asthma does not require any medication and can be fully reversed by the Buteyko Method. Unfortunately, as explained later, standard drug therapy for mild asthma is one of the main reasons that asthma becomes progressively worse.

The Buteyko Method can also help asthmatics who have moderate asthma (i.e. no more than three full-scale asthma attacks during the day and one at night) and also those with severe asthma. The method can prevent repeated acute conditions without medication. It allows for rapid reduction of medication administered as part of the standard asthma treatment, and in most cases, leads to the elimination of all medication.

Typically, a patient will notice significant and lasting improvement in symptoms within one or two weeks after starting the exercises, eventually leading to a life free of symptoms and drugs. The Buteyko Method also provides immediate relief (within one or two minutes) by stopping coughing, whistling, wheezing, shortness of breath (the first sign of an attack), congested nose, etc., without medication. However, as stressed above, successful application of the method requires that the patient practice it conscientiously.

Theoretical Basis

The Buteyko Method is based on a new understanding of the way asthma develops. It is known from basic physiology that one of the main causes of bronchospasm in the lungs is the low level of CO_2 in alveolar air. This causes excessive tension in the smooth muscles of the bronchi, leading to constriction of the bronchi and the feeling of breathlessness. The first scientist to discover this was the Ukrainian medical doctor K. P. Buteyko, who worked in the Siberian branch of the USSR Academy of Medical Science (Institute of Experimental Biology and Medicine, Novosibirsk) and who described this phenomenon in 1962. He proposed a fundamentally new drug-free treatment regime, which was able to increase the level of CO_2 in the lungs back to normal medical levels. This allows the smooth muscles in the walls of the bronchioles to relax, thus avoiding bronchospasms, opening up the airways, and thereby preventing asthma attacks.

If there is a deficiency of CO_2 in the alveolar air the only way to prevent excessive tension (hypertonicity) in the smooth muscles of the bronchi is by taking medication. However, the drugs merely treat the symptoms; if they are stopped, the symptoms will reappear. The underlying cause of asthma is low CO_2 in alveolar air. The Buteyko Method seeks to correct this deficiency by normalizing breathing functions. Evidence of the effectiveness of the method is found in the many former asthmatics in Russia who have lived over 30 years without asthma attacks by following Dr. Buteyko's approach.

Asthma—A Defense Mechanism

The Buteyko Method explains bronchial asthma as a physiological defense mechanism rather than a disease. In order to adequately meet our metabolic needs, there has to be a close match between metabolic activity and ventilation of the lungs. This results in a normal level of CO_2 in the cells, the blood, and in the air of the lungs.

If the metabolic activity is too low for the airflow, or if the airflow is greater than is needed for metabolism, there will be a shortage of CO_2 in the cells, the blood, and in the air of the lungs. Without CO_2, metabolism could not occur. With low CO_2, various systems, such as the immune system, degenerate and become dysfunctional. Under these circumstances, there are two possible outcomes for the organism: it dies or it tries to prevent the excessive loss of CO_2. There are many mechanisms for conserving CO_2 levels. Bronchospasms are one of these mechanisms. Narrowing of the bronchi is an attempt to prevent the loss of CO_2 from the lungs. It follows that asthma is not a disease but simply a physiological response to prevent further loss of CO_2. In this sense, asthma should be viewed in a positive light, as a protective mechanism with real benefit to the asthmatic.[1]

The Hyperventilation Provocation Test

Asthma is not the only response mechanism to low CO2. There are significant differences between individual responses due to genetic disposition. For example, some people develop asthma as a result of low CO2; others suffer from circulatory or neurological disorders. A person's particular predisposition can be tested by monitoring the symptoms provoked through deliberate over-breathing for a limited period of time. By monitoring the first symptoms that occur during this test, you can identify the main mechanism that protects the body from an excessive loss of CO2. Any disease connected to this specific protective mechanism is likely to be dangerous to your health. For example, if an asthmatic experiences a blood vessel spasm as the first symptom during the hyperventilation provocation test, then diseases which are related to the cramping of the blood vessels are even more dangerous than the asthma.

Buteyko's clinical staff in Russia ask their patients to hyperventilate in an attempt to produce or intensify their symptoms. The results of this test invariably convince patients that hyperventilation really is the cause of their disorders and motivates them to apply themselves to the therapy more diligently. It is important to note that this test could be dangerous and must only be done in the presence of a medical practitioner.[2]

---

[1] Indeed, this is why historically asthmatics have a reputation for living long lives. Their asthma effectively protects them from excessive hyperventilation.

[2] Arteries and arterioles have smooth muscles inside their walls just like bronchioles. When arterial CO2 is very low, these smooth muscles can spasm, leading to a narrowing of the vessels. This reduces blood flow and increases blood pressure. The reduced blood flow is partially responsible for the fainting that sometimes occurs during hyperventilation. It can also cause migraines, headaches, and angina, because too little blood reaches the heart and brain. These are some examples of possible symptoms that can arise if you do the hyperventilation provocation test.

The Development of Asthma and Conventional Therapy

Standard modern treatment for chronic bronchitis can lead to the development of bronchial asthma. This may happen during the first six months following a deterioration in a bronchitis. Doctors use antibiotics when a patient's condition deteriorates because this is the most aggressive treatment method available. However, chronic bronchitis cannot be treated with antibiotics indefinitely. After one or two courses of antibiotics the patient may start to experience episodes of breathlessness. Doctors then prescribe drugs normally used for bronchial asthma. As a result, a patient will suffer from increasing breathlessness and become dependent on drugs to treat bronchial asthma. This is the beginning of the development of asthma in a patient. We estimate that some 60 to 70 percent of bronchial asthma is the result of current treatment methods for other diseases, especially treatments for chronic bronchitis. The Buteyko Method allows us to reverse chronic bronchitis in most cases without resorting to antibiotics.

As paradoxical as it may sound, the standard modern drug therapy for asthma is one of the main reasons for the growing prevalence of asthma in many countries today. As previously explained, bronchospasms are a defense mechanism to prevent loss of CO_2 from the lungs. Using drugs to prevent bronchospasm means that we are trying to remove a protective mechanism designed to conserve CO_2. Suppression of this mechanism leads to more CO_2 loss and stronger bronchospasms once the effect of the drugs wears off. The result is that the asthma condition worsens. Unlike most other diseases, asthma is simply a survival mechanism.

CO2 Levels in the Lungs and in the Blood

This section is not essential reading in order to master Buteyko breathing exercises. It is included mainly for the benefit of the more technically minded who are often puzzled by an apparent contradiction concerning the method. The aim of the method is to decrease lung ventilation in order to increase alveolar CO_2. However, many asthmatics have high blood CO_2. This leads doctors to recommend the opposite—increased lung ventilation—in order to reduce blood CO2, because the high CO2 is due to insufficient ventilation. However, increased breathing will reduce alveolar CO2 and usually provokes a bronchospasm. This presents a dilemma for doctors.

In 1962, Dr. Buteyko, for the first time in the history of medicine, resolved this paradox. He explained that the difference between blood CO2 and lung CO2 that exists in some asthmatics is caused by damage to lung tissue resulting in a deterioration of the gas exchange process in the lung. In this case, the increased ventilation causes a deficiency only in the lung CO2 resulting in hypertonicity of the smooth muscle in the walls of the bronchi, provoking bronchospasms.

The following diagram approximately represents the gas exchange in the lungs with normal indices of CO2 and O2 in alveolar air and blood.

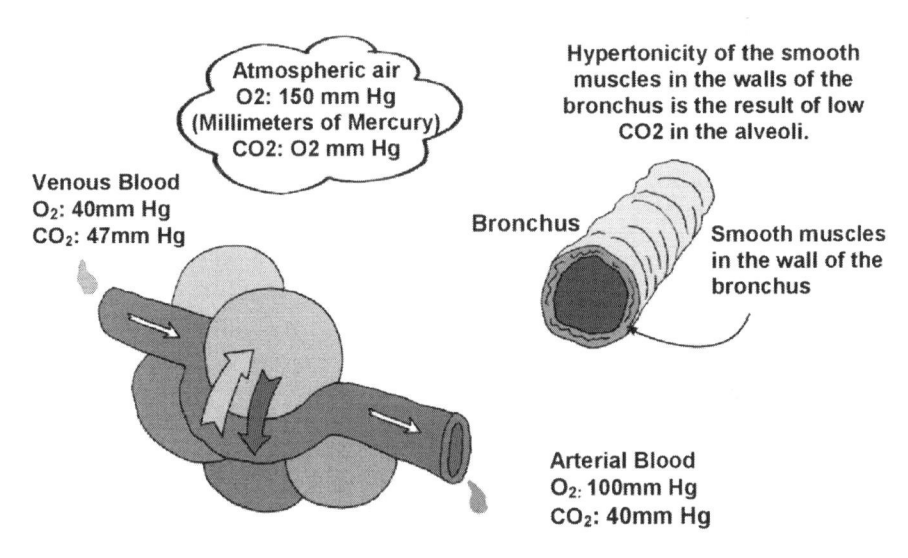

Atmospheric air
O2: 150 mm Hg
(Millimeters of Mercury)
CO2: 02 mm Hg

Venous Blood
O_2: 40mm Hg
CO_2: 47mm Hg

Hypertonicity of the smooth muscles in the walls of the bronchus is the result of low CO2 in the alveoli.

Bronchus

Smooth muscles in the wall of the bronchus

Arterial Blood
O_2: 100mm Hg
CO_2: 40mm Hg

But in asthma these indices are not normal. Usually, asthmatics have consistently very low levels of CO2 in alveolar air, while the CO2 in the blood can be low, normal or high, depending on the severity of the asthma. The consistently low level of alveolar CO2 is a result of chronic alveolar hyperventilation. The high level of CO2 in the blood is a result of destroyed or damaged lung tissue, resulting in a deterioration of the gas exchange process in the lung. The following illustrates how alveolar and blood CO2 can vary in asthmatics.

1. Normal CO2

In healthy individuals or in individuals with early stage asthma, alveolar and blood CO2 are the same. This assumes that the lung tissues are normal and that a normal gas exchange takes place through the alveolar membranes.

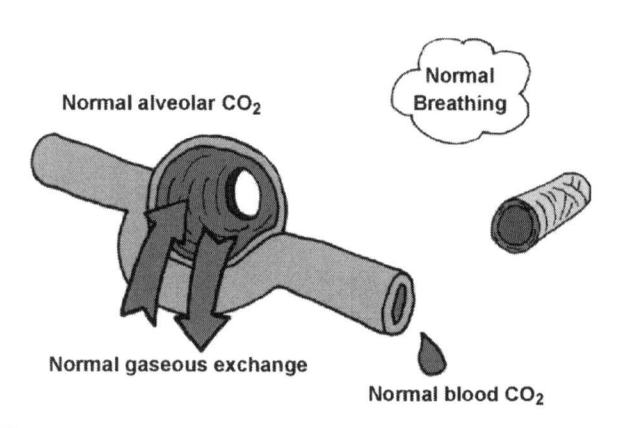

2. Low CO2

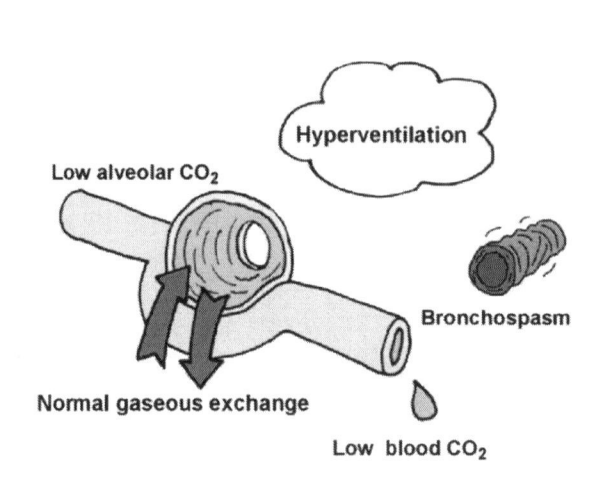

Alveolar membranes are normal, while both alveolar and blood CO2 are low. In healthy individuals the alveolar CO2 level is around 40mm Hg. It is never this high in asthmatics. The reason for the low level of CO2 found in the lungs is chronic hyperventilation.

3. High CO2

In severe asthma, alveolar CO2 is always very low. CO2 in the blood is high in severe asthma and occasionally in mild-to-moderate asthma. This results from destroyed tissue in the lungs and a deterioration of gas exchange in the lung. Pulmonary emphysema and pneumosclerosis can often cause arteriovenous shunting in the lung. With this condition, the destruction of the lung tissue in some areas prevents normal gas exchange, resulting in the venous blood from these areas, with its high CO2 and low O2 content, effectively being shunted back into the arteries.

Alveolar CO2 should be measured at the end of a normal exhalation. It often happens that end tidal CO2 measurements appear to show higher than usual CO2 levels in alveolar air. This happens when there is an unnaturally long exhalation. In this event, the air closest to the blood, which is richer in CO2 enters the gas analyzer, which will show a higher percentage of CO2 in the alveoli than the average value. For this reason, it is important to measure CO2 correctly after a normal exhalation, especially if there is normal gas exchange in the lungs.

4. Changes of CO2 and O2 in the alveoli, in the blood and in the cells

The level of CO2 in the alveolar air is important. One of the main characteristics of bronchial asthma is excessive tension of the smooth muscles of the bronchi (hypertonicity). This is the result of low alveolar CO2 and cause a bronchospasm. If you are aiming to prevent an asthma attack, you need to have a normal level of CO2 in the lungs. At the same time, CO2 in the blood can be high or normal. Bronchospasm and asthma attacks are not dependent on the level of CO2 in the blood.

According to Dr. Buteyko, there are two main reasons for the low level of CO2 in the lungs of asthmatics:

1. "Chronic alveolar hyperventilation" or "excessive breathing." In other words, too much air flows through the lungs, removing

excessive amounts of CO2. This causes the alveolar air to be depleted of CO2.

2. Low metabolic activity, resulting in low CO 2 production.

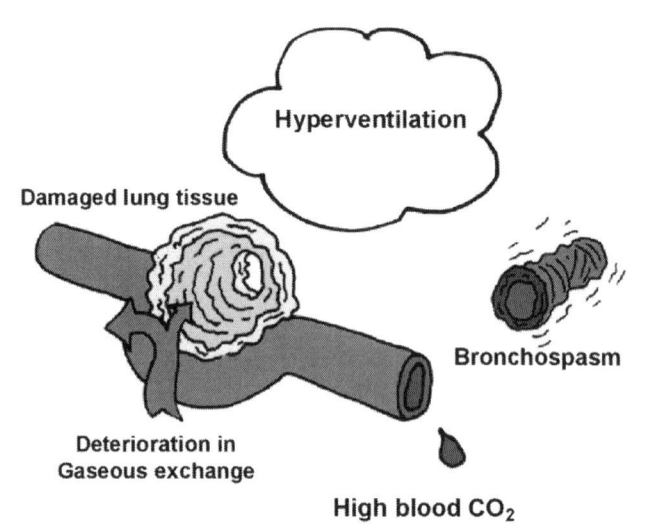

Hyperventilation

Damaged lung tissue

Bronchospasm

Deterioration in Gaseous exchange

High blood CO_2

This following graph shows the approximate changes of CO2 and O2 in the alveoli, in the blood, and in the cells, depending on the changes in lung tissue and the deterioration of gas exchange in the lungs.

BREATHE TO HEAL

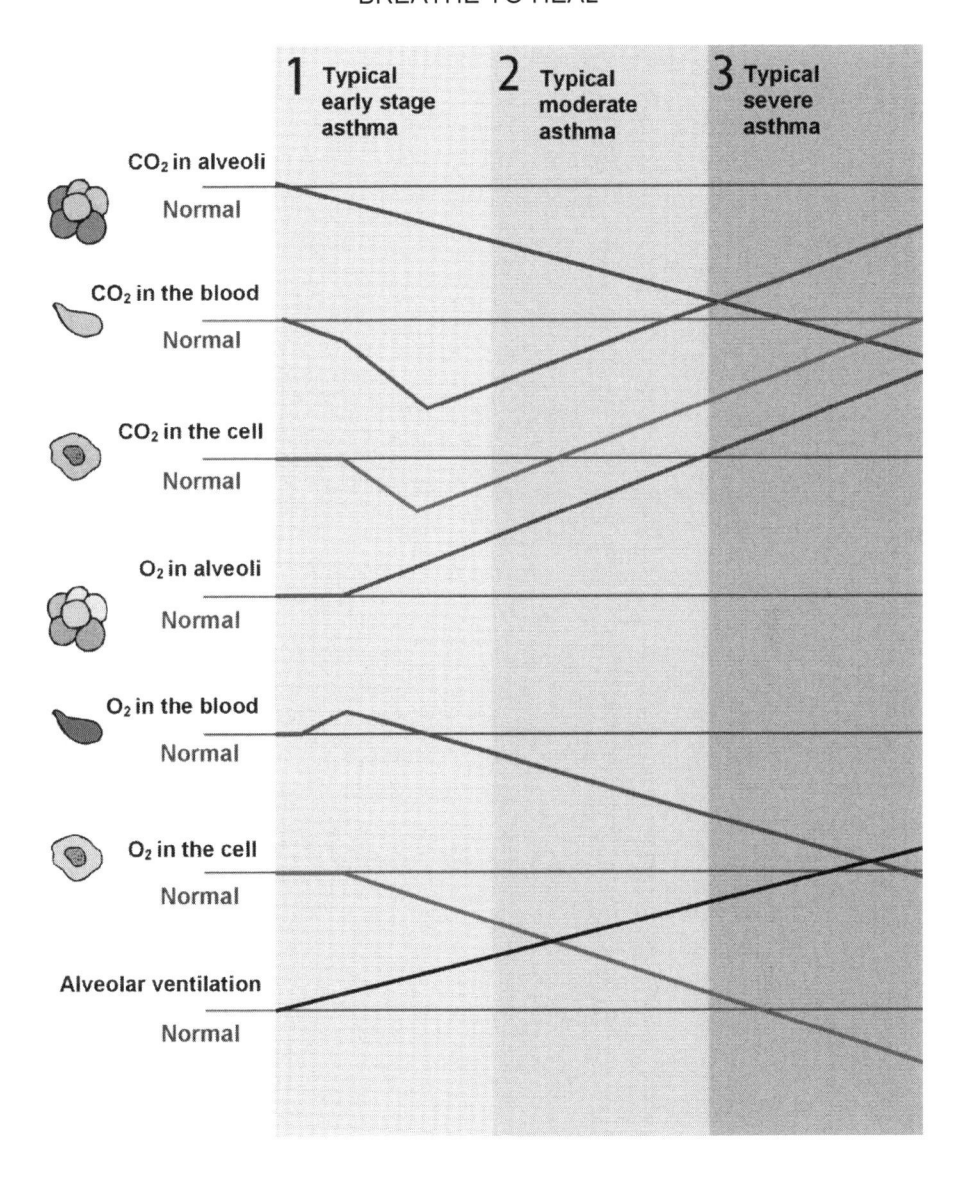

| | **1** Typical early stage asthma | **2** Typical moderate asthma | **3** Typical severe asthma |

CO_2 in alveoli
Normal

CO_2 in the blood
Normal

CO_2 in the cell
Normal

O_2 in alveoli
Normal

O_2 in the blood
Normal

O_2 in the cell
Normal

Alveolar ventilation
Normal

5. Three ways to stabilize the level of CO2 in the alveolar air

1. Conscious control: Reduce the airflow by using conscious control with special breathing exercises. These allow you to match the ventilation of the lungs to the needs of your metabolism. The main types of Buteyko exercises are described in detail in this book. All the exercises are designed to reduce the depth of breathing, with variations between exercises adapted to different situations.

2. Exercise: Increase muscle activity through exercise. This will increase CO2 as one of the products of metabolism. This is the more natural way, but it is very important to control and limit the rate at which air flows through your lungs while exercising. If you are already hyperventilating, it is not possible to increase the level of CO2 by exercising because breathing is likely to increase more quickly than the CO2 produced, thus provoking an asthma attack. The breathing exercises will help you match your lung ventilation to your metabolic needs during exercise (see "How to reverse asthma using physical exercise.").

3. Identify Causes: Identify and eliminate any causes of excessive breathing. There are many factors, such as overeating, over-sleeping, excessive breathing while speaking, prolonged stress and other habits and circumstances likely to increase breathing. This will lead to lower CO2 levels in the lungs, which in turn may provoke a bronchospasm and an acute asthma attack. If your baseline level of CO2 in the alveolar air is already low, any further reduction in CO2, caused by overeating or over-sleeping, will intensify deep breathing and may provoke an asthma attack. Therefore, it is important to learn to control your breathing in any situation; for example, when you sleep, drive a car, dance, make a declaration of love or simply visit a bank. The Buteyko Method provides advice on diet and lifestyle habits. This advice should be adapted to the circumstances of the individual and is best provided by a Breathing Normalization Specialist. It should also be noted that once CO2 levels are restored to normal, factors relating to diet, sleep, etc. become less important.

Part 2: Breathing Awareness and Measurements

Mindfulness of Breathing

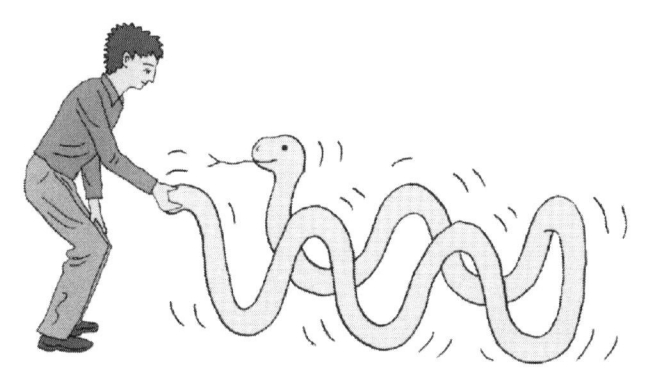

The small clouds show the volume of air inhaled and exhaled. The curves of the snake illustrate the process of inhalation (breathing in) and exhalation (breathing out).

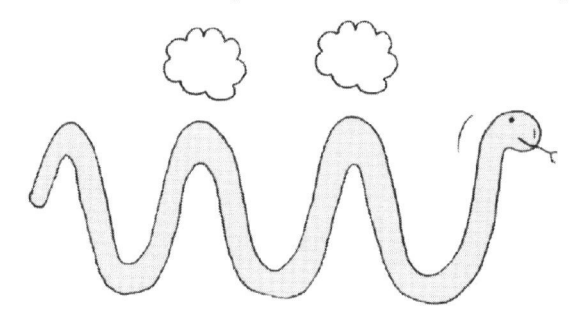

Breathing

In order to help you do the breathing exercises, we would like to introduce you at this point to the Breathing Snake.

Breathing can conveniently be represented by the undulations of a snake. The snake's symbolic significance also encompasses Dr. Buteyko's own philosophy on breathing: that it is a physiological process, which needs to be respected and treated with great sensitivity, as if it were a living thing.

Gentle or normal, breathing is a fundamental requirement for a long and healthy life. Over-breathing is the basis of many diseases. So we

Part 2: Breathing Awareness and Measurements by Andrey Novozhilov, MD

can regard our breath as an enemy when it is excessive and as a friend when it is normal or gentle. We also use colors to illustrate the volume of breathing. Red stands for over-breathing, blue for gentle breathing, and yellow and green for those breathing states in between.

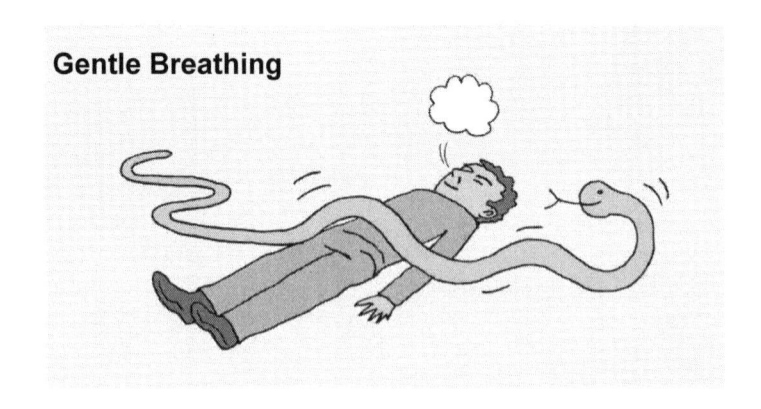

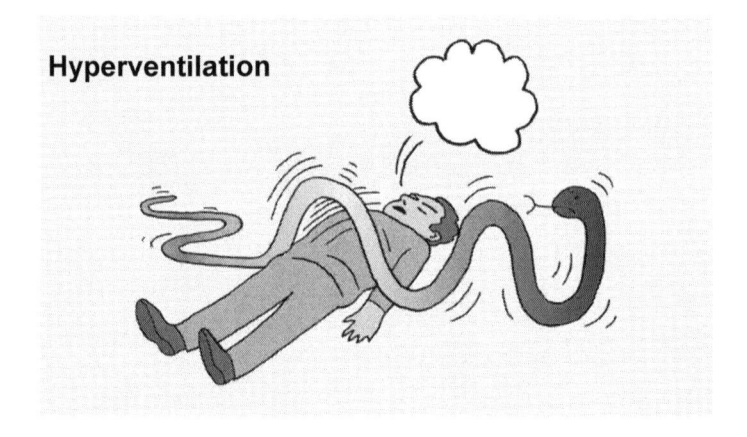

Gentle Breathing

Hyperventilation

BREATHE TO HEAL

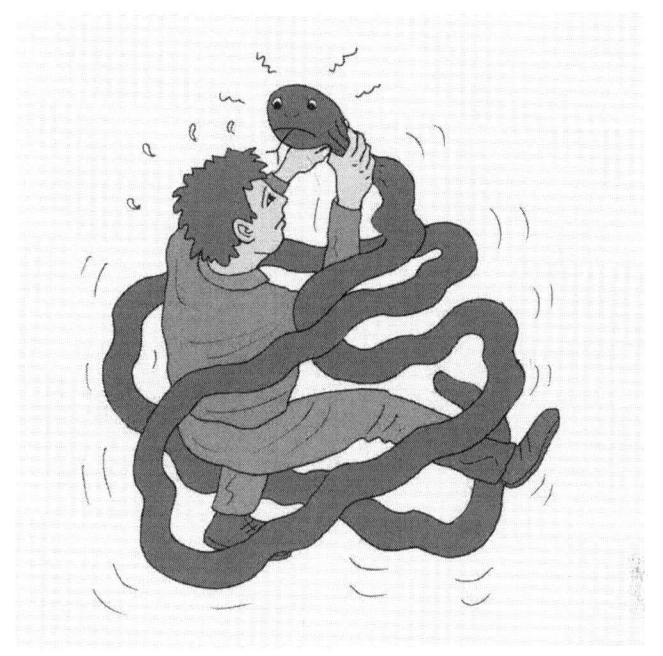

Rehabilitation of breathing should never be a struggle.

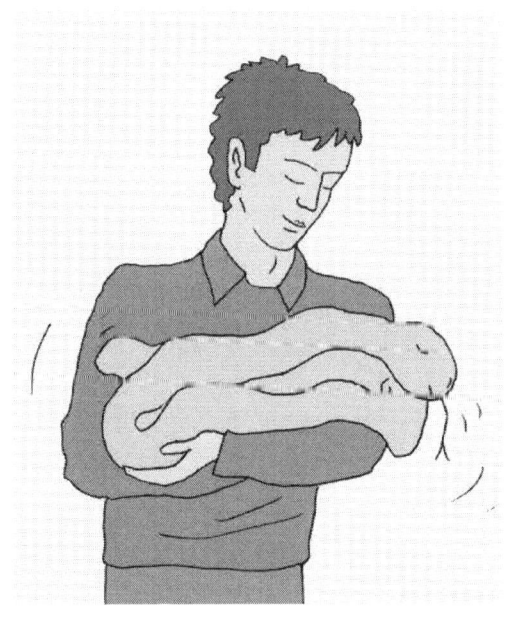

Instead, breathing should be regarded as something living and scared to be cherished and nurtured, like a baby.

Various Breathing Measurements

Dr. Buteyko developed three forms of breathing measurements—please see their descriptions below:

1. Control Pause:
The length of time you can hold your breath so that on resumption of breathing you immediately assume the pattern of breathing you had before the breath-hold.

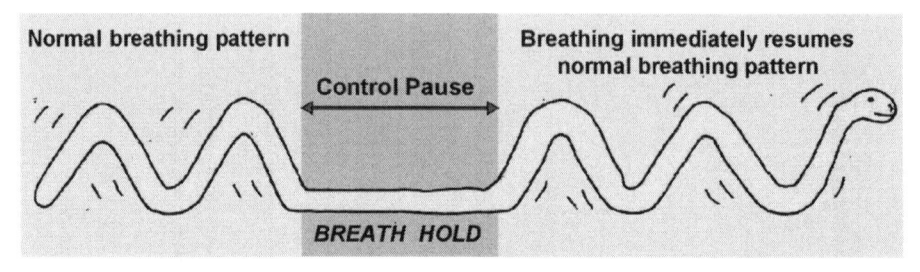

Control Pause

2. Positive Maximum Pause:
The maximum length of time you can hold your breath comfortably, and on resumption of breathing force your breathing into the pattern of breathing you had before the breath-hold.

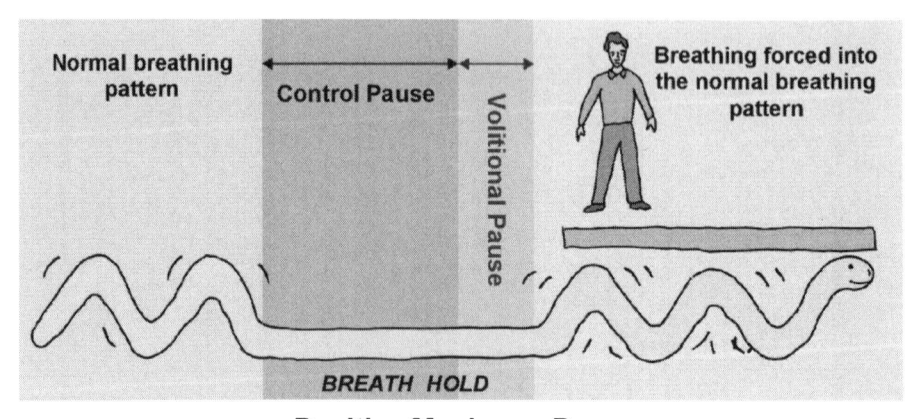

Positive Maximum Pause

3. Negative Maximum Pause (or Absolute Maximum Pause):

The absolutely longest period you can manage to hold your breath, where on resumption of breathing it is no longer possible to force your breathing into the pattern before the breath-hold.

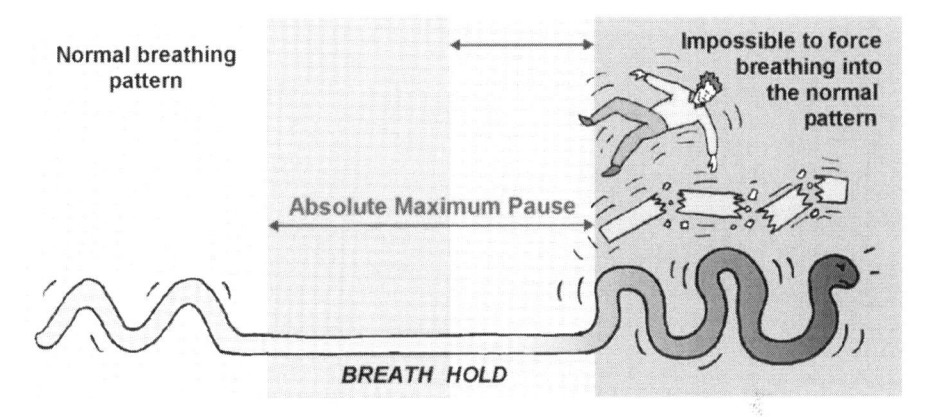

Negative or Absolute Maximum Pause

About Control Pause:

Even though Dr. Buteyko mostly used Positive Maximum Pause for his work, the measurement of Control Pause became the most common, since it is the easiest for beginners. In this book, I will mostly use the term Positive Maximum Pause occasionally referring to Control Pause. Generally, there is no problem in using these terms interchangeably.

A short definition of the term *Control Pause* is "the time that you can hold your breath until you feel the first impulse to breathe in again." On resumption of breathing you must be able to assume the pattern of breathing you had just before you started to hold your breath. Just remember that Control Pause is always shorter than Positive Maximum Pause (Dr. Buteyko referred to it as "Maximum Pause".)

Dr. Buteyko developed Control Pause/ Positive Maximum Pause as a simple and reliable measure of the CO2 level in the lungs. When he started to develop the method, there was no need to use these breathing measurements because Dr. Buteyko had a well-equipped laboratory at his disposal and instruments to measure CO2. However, when his laboratory was destroyed, he had to find a new simple way of measuring CO2. So he developed the concept of the Positive Maximum Pause and later Control Pause. Maximum Pause is a more complex way to measure breathing; therefore, Control Pause as a simpler measurement is normally used in the beginning of the breathing normalization process. As I already mentioned, in this book I will use both types of measurements.

Below I will explain in detail how to measure your Control Pause. Positive Maximum Pause is measured in the same way with the exception that a hold after exhalation is slightly longer, and therefore, could be mildly uncomfortable.

In order to measure your breathing, you will need a stopwatch or a clock that has a second hand to count the seconds.

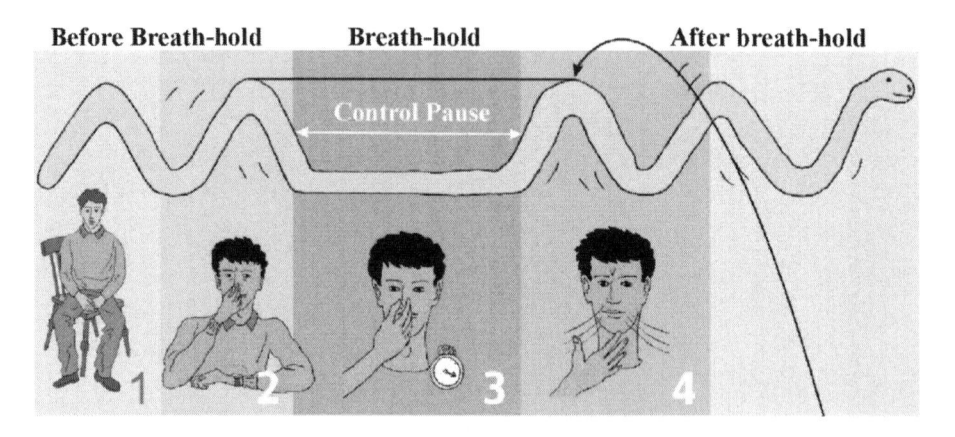

How to measure Control Pause:

1. Assume the correct posture, with a straight back.

2. After exhaling normally, hold your nose with your fingers.

3. Start your stopwatch or look at the second hand of your watch. Hold your breath until you feel the first need to breathe again. The entire breath-hold must be completely effortless. The duration of this breath-hold is called the "Control Pause."

4. As soon as you feel the first need to breathe again, release your nose and resume breathing. The depth of the first inhalation must be as it was when you started holding your breath.

The most important thing to remember:
The depth of the first breath at the end of the CP should not be deeper than it was just before you started the breath-hold.

Possible mistakes in measuring Control Pause:

- You continue to hold your breath, with some effort, beyond the point where you feel the first urge to breathe. By doing so, your breath-hold will be longer than your true CP.

- You measure your CP immediately after doing breathing exercises. This is likely to lead to measuring a shorter breath-hold than your true CP because right after doing exercises you experience a slight shortage of air. You should, therefore, wait three to five minutes after doing Buteyko breathing exercises before taking your CP.

- You alter your breathing in any way (including doing Buteyko breathing exercises) before measuring your CP. This will result in a false reading. You should measure your CP under standard conditions. This means that you should measure your CP when you are breathing normally without paying any particular attention to how you are breathing.

- You measure your CP too soon after doing physical exercise. This is likely to produce an inaccurate and low measurement. After physical exercise, it is particularly important to wait until normal breathing is restored (around 10 to 15 minutes; however, in some cases it can be up to an hour) before you measure your CP.

The Morning Control Pause:
The Control Pause you measure in the morning after a night's sleep is especially significant. This is referred to as the Morning CP. It is a more reliable index of health than your CP taken at other times because you cannot control breathing during sleep. It is, therefore, a measure of your natural state of breathing. CPs taken during the day can vary significantly; for example, before dinner you may have a CP

of 20, but after dinner, it could drop to 5. Which of these is the real CP? Also, CPs taken immediately after vigorous exercise will be lower than before exercising. It is, therefore, desirable to use the Morning CP as the baseline reading. If you have a CP of 10 to 20 seconds during the day, but your Morning CP is only 5 seconds, then your genuine CP is 5 seconds. Higher CPs measured during the day are less significant.

When people are told that asthma attacks will stop when they have a CP greater than 20 seconds, it means that they must have a Morning CP of more than 20 seconds. It is not important what CP or Positive Maximum Pause (PMP) they have during the day. Often asthmatics have a CP of 30 to 40 seconds throughout the day and PMP of 60-80 seconds but they still suffer from asthma attacks because their Morning CP is less than 20 seconds. Of course, if their Morning CP is 20 seconds, their Morning PMP should be much higher: for example, it could be 40 seconds.

Part 3: Buteyko Breathing Exercises

Understand How To Do The Exercises

The main aim of all Buteyko breathing exercises is to reduce the volume of air that flows through the lungs every minute (the Minute Volume is described on the next page). This enables CO2 to build back up to normal, thereby stopping and preventing bronchospasms.

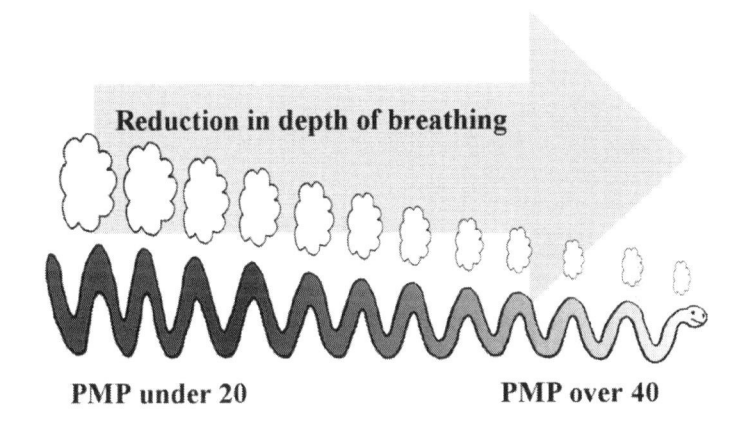

Reduction in depth of breathing

PMP under 20   **PMP over 40**

When this aim is realized, metabolism and the immune system will automatically revert to normal. For example, if your Morning PMP is more than 40, you will know that you are free of viral and other infections.

The Buteyko Method aims to change the volume of breathing, not the breathing rate. You, therefore, need to reduce the depth of every inhalation to normal. Nevertheless, there is a connection between the volume and frequency of breathing:

- Excessive and rapid breathing tend to go together. If an asthmatic has a PMP of five to 10 scoonds this will usually be associated with a respiration rate of 20 to 50 breaths per minute.

- A person with a PMP of 60 seconds typically will take only three to five breaths per minute and automatically leave a short pause between breaths. This automatic pause can extend to 10 to 20 seconds with a breathing rate of three to five breaths per minute.

- The first automatic pause in breathing will appear when you have a Morning PMP of at least 20 seconds, which means that periodically you automatically hold your breath for one second after exhalation.

It is important to reduce the volume of breathing rather than the breathing rate because:

- If you have a well-developed sensitivity to your breathing process, you will feel the natural need to stop breathing for one to two seconds, especially during Exercise 1. ("How to reduce the depth of breathing through relaxation"). You should not try to suppress such pauses.

- You cannot reduce the airflow by changing the respiration rate, as this will deepen your breathing. The Buteyko breathing exercises aim just to change the depth of breathing. The frequency will change naturally and automatically.

"To reduce the depth of breathing" essentially means that the volume of air inhaled during and after the exercises is less than the volume of air before the exercises. See the following illustration.

Minute Volume

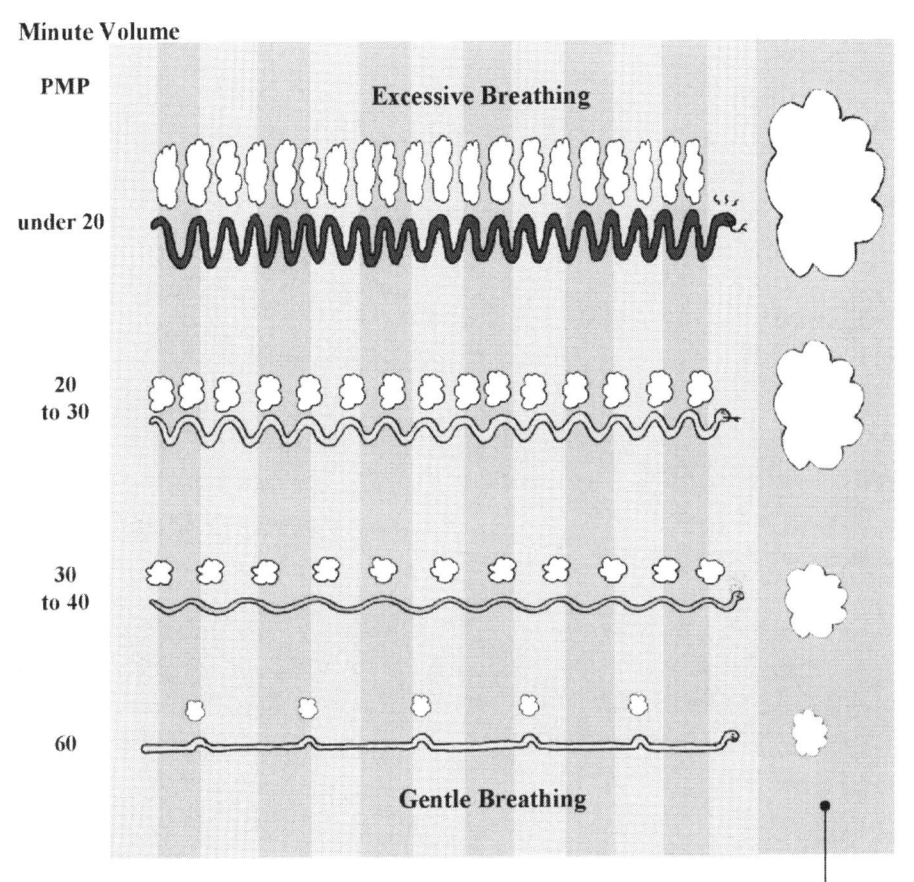

PMP	
under 20	Excessive Breathing
20 to 30	
30 to 40	
60	Gentle Breathing

Total volume of air breathed in and out in one minute

When and for how long you should do the Buteyko breathing exercises?

If you are suffering from asthma symptoms, or experiencing other symptoms of hyperventilation-related diseases, you should carry out the breathing exercises until the symptoms disappear. The particular type of exercise you choose is not important as long as it enables you to reduce the volume of your breathing. You should feel free to experiment to find the exercises that suit you best.

For example, when you have a headache, you should establish a slight but comfortable feeling of air shortage by relaxing until the headache disappears. If the feeling of air shortage is too strong, the headache will become more severe for at least 5 to 10 minutes before it subsides.

What to do if you are not experiencing symptoms?
If you do not have any symptoms, you should do the Buteyko breathing exercises until your CP is at least five seconds higher than it was when you started the exercise. You need a difference of at least five seconds to ensure that your CP really has risen. Smaller differences could be due to measurement error. Remember to only measure your CP three to five minutes after doing breathing exercises, not immediately after. This is because right after exercising, you automatically feel a slight air shortage, and your CP will be lower. Do not worry about this, but have a rest and resume normal breathing without feeling any air shortage. Measure your CP again after your breathing has settled.

It is not important how much time you spend doing your breathing exercises. It is much more important to ensure that the CP after the exercise is higher than it was before. This is a fundamental principle of the Breathing Normalization. You will only conquer asthma if you can raise your CP.

If you need five minutes to increase your CP, it means that five minutes is enough for you at one sitting. As a rule, your CP will decrease after roughly one or two hours. You should then start to increase it again with another exercise.

You may perform Buteyko breathing exercises in many short bursts of three to five minutes throughout the day, with rests in between. The point is not to spend any particular amount of time on these exercises; it's all about making sure that the CP increases, no matter how long it takes.

Consult your Breathing Normalization Specialist
Rehabilitation of your breathing is not to be undertaken casually. Successful application of the Buteyko Method is greatly assisted if you are able to learn the method under the supervision of an experienced Buteyko practitioner. This is especially true if you suffer from severe

asthma. As explained earlier, this book is written in order to explain clearly how the main exercises should be performed in order to satisfy the demand for reliable information about the practical application of the technique. However, there is no guarantee that you will be able to interpret the exercises correctly or know how to adapt them to your particular circumstances. It is important, therefore, that if you feel your health worsening or find that you are provoking asthma attacks, you should stop the exercises immediately and seek guidance from a practitioner.

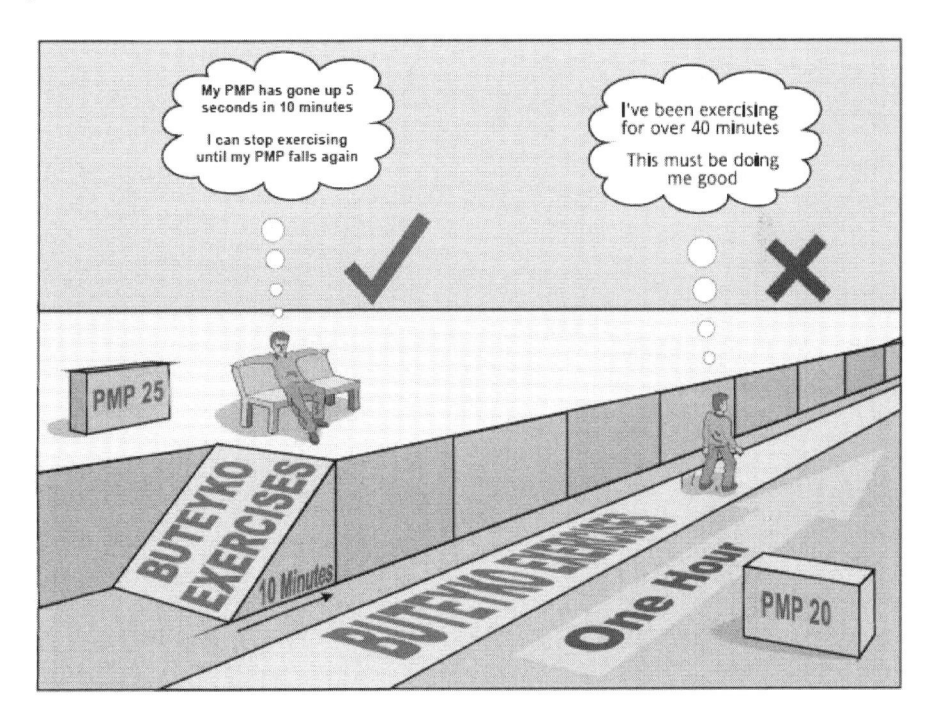

[Figure: Two scenarios comparing Buteyko exercises. Left (✓): "My PMP has gone up 5 seconds in 10 minutes. I can stop exercising until my PMP falls again" — PMP 25, Buteyko Exercises 10 Minutes. Right (✗): "I've been exercising for over 40 minutes. This must be doing me good" — Buteyko Exercises One Hour, PMP 20.]

Most of the Buteyko exercises are based on an ability to sense your breathing. A Buteyko Breathing Normalization Specialist will teach you how this is done and how to reduce your volume of breathing easily and comfortably at any place and in any situation. If you cannot see and feel how you breathe, you are likely to start increasing your airflow instead of reducing it. Such attempts may then result in an asthma attack. In these cases, your practitioner will help you adopt a suitable alternative exercise. A practitioner will also provide advice regarding other factors related to diet (such as eating too much) and other habits (talking a lot in the wrong way, over-sleeping, not being able to relax, etc.), which may increase hyperventilation and provoke asthma attacks.

Once you have increased your level of CO_2 to normal medical levels, your metabolism will automatically normalize and your symptoms caused by hyperventilation will disappear. You will then be able to lead a normal life being free of asthma attacks.

How can you tell that you are doing the exercises correctly?
You are doing the exercises correctly if:

- You are able to overcome the asthma symptoms

- Your PMP or CP increases

- You are able to induce a feeling of air shortage when you reduce the depth of every inhalation through conscious control. This feeling is the main sign that the airflow has been reduced. The level of air shortage may be either large or small. Establishing a slight feeling of air hunger should always be a comfortable experience.

Different breathing exercises produce varying levels of the feeling of air shortage. The extent of this feeling depends on the particular exercise being performed.

Exercises done during muscular activity can develop any level of air shortage, small or big. If you do the exercises without muscular activity, you should only develop a feeling of very mild air shortage, and this should remain comfortable. However, if you perform breathing exercises while engaging in physical activity, you can develop even a strong feeling of air shortage.

Choice of Exercise
All Buteyko breathing exercises described in this book are intended to reduce the volume of breathing, with variations between exercises designed for different situations. The choice of exercise is your decision, depending on your circumstances and what you find suits

you best. The best exercise is one that enables you to increase your CP or PMP significantly.

There is an important distinction between the three approaches described under Exercise # 1 and the other breathing exercises. Exercise # 1 achieves a more sustained reduction of breathing through relaxation. The other exercises depend on willpower—exerting control on the breathing muscles to reduce the depth of breathing. The use of conscious control increases CO2 over relatively short periods of time and does not result in the same lasting reduction of airflow and altered breathing pattern as is possible using Exercise # 1. It is, therefore, necessary to repeat often the exercises that cultivate a shortage of air until your CP/PMP has stabilized at a higher level.

While reducing airflow through relaxation might be the ideal approach, some individuals with a low level of CO2 have problems in sensing their breathing. They find it difficult to achieve the degree of mental and physical relaxation necessary to induce a significant reduction in airflow. In such cases, they should try one of the other exercises until their PMP is at least 20 seconds. As their PMP improves, they should find it progressively easier to practice a variant of Exercise # 1.

It is also quite common for people to have the opposite problem; in other words, finding it difficult to reduce breathing through conscious control. Problems can arise if too much effort is used to reduce breathing. This can be uncomfortable and can result in an increase in airflow because of tension and anxiety. In such cases, it is important to concentrate on finding ways to relax the mind and body, especially the breathing muscles. An experienced practitioner will be able to help you to choose the approach that is likely to suit you best.

All breathing exercises should be practiced diligently until the morning Positive Maximum Pause is consistently above 40 seconds.

Key points about breath-holds
The CP is a reliable measure of your state of breathing and health and plays a central role in the Buteyko Method.

As will be seen in later sections, breath-holds longer than the CP are used in some breathing exercises in order to raise the level of CO2. However, they do not provide any useful scientific information like the breathing measurements (CP and PMP) do.

If you hold your breath for too long you will find it impossible to control your breathing when you end the breath-hold. It is an important principle of the Buteyko breathing exercises that when these involve breath-holds longer than the CP, you should always be able to force your breathing immediately afterwards back into your normal pattern. Otherwise, your breathing can become disordered and you risk increasing, rather than reducing, hyperventilation.

Exercise # 1: How to reduce the volume of breathing through relaxation

The objective of Exercise # 1 is to reduce breathing, and therefore, increase CO2 in the lungs through relaxation and the development of an acute awareness of how you breathe. This is so fundamental to the Buteyko approach that three different approaches to breath reduction through relaxation are described below.

All these approaches have the same objective to reduce breathing through relaxation. They all depend on a quiet mind focused on the breathing process, leading to profound physical and mental relaxation and a reduced airflow. The first approach develops an acute awareness of breathing. The second approach suggests you imagine that your breathing is slowing down without the exertion of any force to reduce breathing. The third approach is similar to the second, but focuses on visualizing the pattern of breathing. A variety of approaches is described, as you may find that one works better for you than another.

These exercises are not as easy as they seem because they require a lot of attention on the breathing process as well as extreme sensitivity to your breathing.

Approach 1: Awareness of the breathing process

The aim of this exercise is to decrease your level of breathing by developing an extensive awareness of your breathing and relaxing the corresponding muscles. It is desirable to adopt the correct posture by sitting comfortably with your back straight. Try to see and feel the process of your breathing. Ask yourself what it is that you feel and see during the inhalation and exhalation process.

Focus on relaxing your body from the head downwards. Pay full attention to relaxing all the muscles involved with inhalation. Concentrate on relaxing the muscles around the diaphragm. This is the area above your stomach, between the navel and breastbone.

Maintain good posture, draw in your stomach a little and feel and see how your ribcage rises a little higher than it did before. Then, relax the upper part of the muscles of your stomach. This will cause the stomach to extend a little.

This exercise will increase your awareness of the volume of air that flows through the lungs. After a period of intense concentration on relaxing and sensing your breathing (10 to 40 minutes), the depth of your breathing will naturally start to decrease until it reaches a new significantly reduced level.

At this point, your CP/PMP should increase by 10 to 20 percent. The time it takes to reduce breathing will depend on your circumstances and the extent to which the breathing muscles become relaxed. There should be no effort involved in this exercise. You should not consciously alter the level of your breathing. Remember, the aim is to reduce breathing through relaxation.

Part 3: Buteyko Breathing Exercises by Andrey Novozhilov, MD

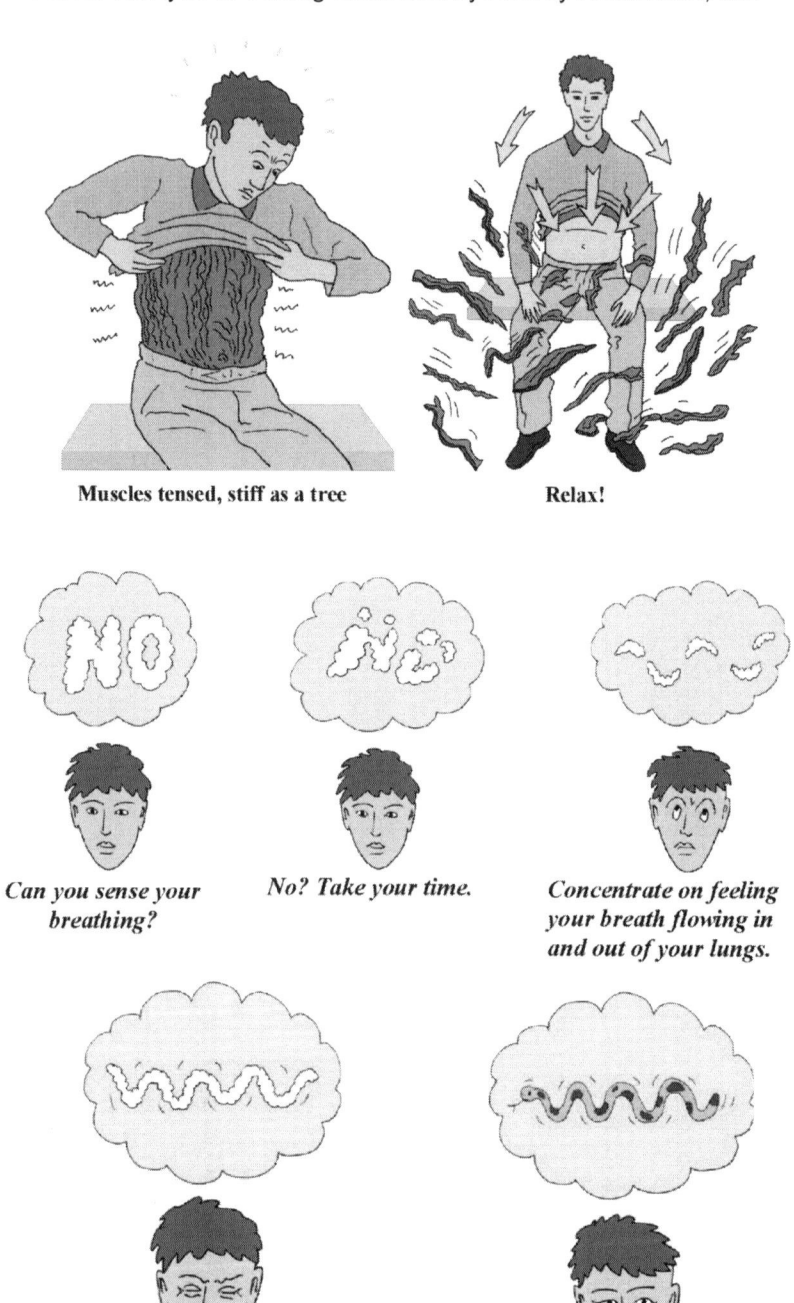

Muscles tensed, stiff as a tree

Relax!

Can you sense your breathing?

No? Take your time.

Concentrate on feeling your breath flowing in and out of your lungs.

That's it! Tune in to the pattern of your breathing

Become very aware of your breathing

Try to do this exercise at all times and in all situations. Be aware of your breathing, and focus at all times on relaxation. It is a good idea to set aside a fixed amount of time each day to sit down for this exercise until you have become proficient at it. Do not be discouraged if you find it hard to relax at first. With practice you will discover how to let go of your breathing muscles to the extent necessary to induce reduced breathing.

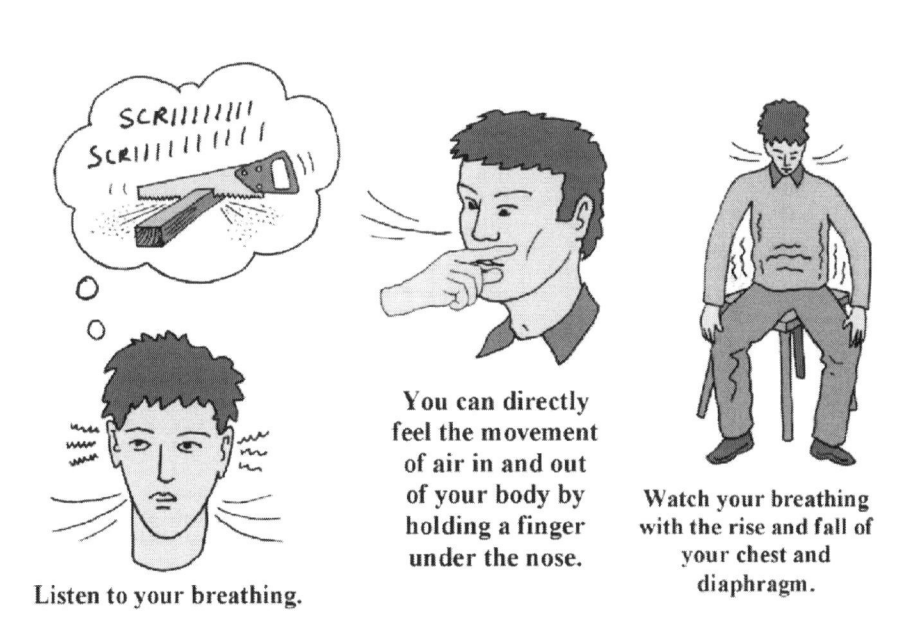

Listen to your breathing.

You can directly feel the movement of air in and out of your body by holding a finger under the nose.

Watch your breathing with the rise and fall of your chest and diaphragm.

Approach 2: Extraordinary sense of well-being

Assume the correct posture by sitting up—back straight, shoulders relaxed. This posture will ensure that the stomach is naturally drawn in without any effort or tension in the abdominal muscles. Do not interfere with your breathing at this stage. This can be difficult because just by adopting this posture the depth of breathing automatically reduces a little. This can make you want to encourage this process further by exerting a degree of conscious control. It is important not to cultivate a feeling of air shortage.

Having assumed this erect posture, try to sense your breathing. What exactly do you feel? Do you feel movement of air in the nose? Do you hear your breathing? Do you see your stomach and chest moving as you breathe?

Now imagine the airflow is reducing a little. You should not try to slow the airflow down through conscious control of your breathing. It should be sufficient simply to imagine a reduction in airflow. Relaxing, sensing your breathing, and imagining—but not forcing—a reduction in airflow should result in a real slight reduction in depth of breathing. You should feel comfortable, calm, at ease and totally relaxed.

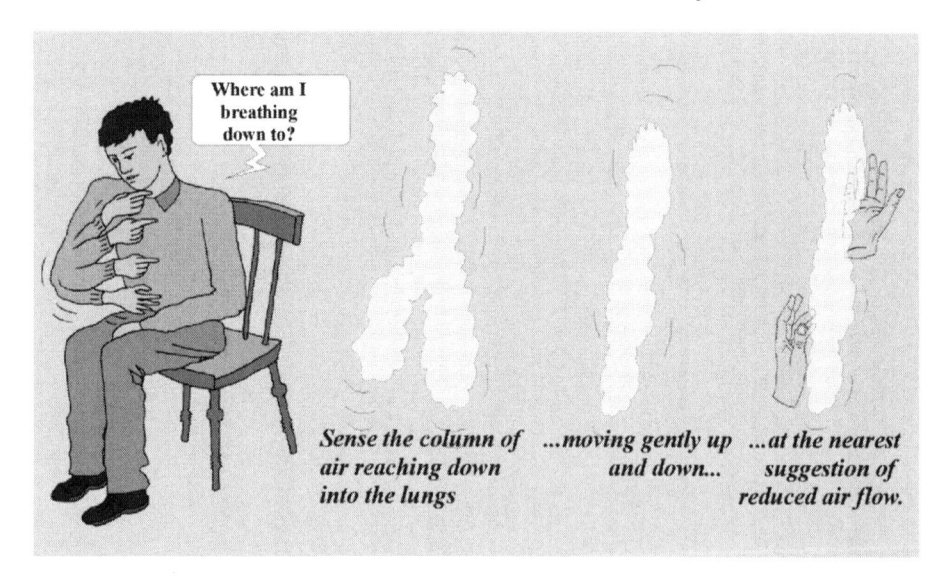

Sense the column of air reaching down into the lungs ...*moving gently up and down*... ...*at the nearest suggestion of reduced air flow.*

Try to sustain this comfortable feeling of slightly reduced airflow for 5 seconds, 10 seconds, 20 seconds, and then longer. If you feel a little tense after 5 to 10 seconds, then you will have lost that comfortable feeling, and you will be breathing more, instead of less. This tension is a result of trying to reduce breathing with effort rather than with relaxation. For this exercise, it is a mistake to reduce breathing by willpower. If this happens, stop your exercise, distract your mind for a minute or two, and start again.

Initially, you may only be able to do this exercise for 5 to 10 seconds. Later, you will be able to do it all day long. This exercise resonates with the words of Lao Tzu (500 BC): "The perfect man breathes as if he is not breathing."

Approach 3: Just hint at reduction of airflow

This exercise aims to decrease your level of breathing by focusing your attention only on the pattern of your breathing.

Take up a correct posture by sitting comfortably with your back straight. Try to visualize, hear and feel your breathing. What do you detect? Do you feel movement of air in your nose? Do you feel movement of your chest or stomach while trying to sense your breathing?

Try to visualize the pattern of your breathing. What is the frequency of your breathing? What is the duration of each inhalation and exhalation? Is your breathing regular and calm, or is it erratic?

You do not need to do arithmetic to calculate the frequency of your breathing, nor do you need to count the duration or every inhalation and exhalation in seconds. However, you do need to develop a sense of the pattern of your breathing. This is important because when your airflow starts to reduce, you need to compare your new pattern with the one you had before the exercise.

Decrease the volume of breathing without any dramatic change in the pattern of breathing.

Breathing pattern before the exercise   Breathing pattern during the exercise

Try to decrease the volume of breathing by imagining that your airflow becomes a little diminished. You should hold this sensation without any dramatic change in the pattern of your breathing. If you sense that the pattern is changing, then you have decreased the volume of breathing too vigorously. If this happens, stop your exercise, distract your mind for a minute or two, and start again. In this exercise, it is a mistake to try to reduce breathing by willpower.

Excessive decrease in the volume of breathing resulting in a dramatic change in the breathing. pattern. This must be avoided.

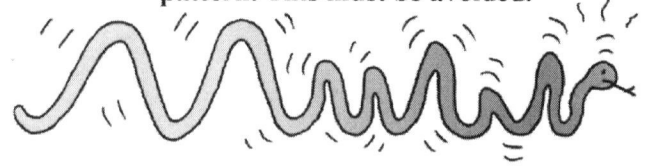

Breathing before   The frequency of breathing is modified.

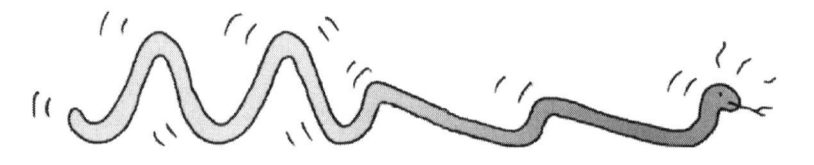

Breathing before   The duration of each inhalation/exhalation is modified.

Notes for Exercise 1 – Approach 1, 2 and 3 (*Possible mistakes*)

Consciously interfering with the breathing process in order to achieve a reduced airflow more quickly. Reduction in depth of breathing through Exercise 1 should arise naturally and automatically as a result of relaxation and thinking about reduced airflow without effort.

- Having, at any point, a feeling of hunger for air. Once your volume of breathing has reduced, this will be a very comfortable feeling which should be easy to sustain.
- Increasing the frequency of your breathing or changing the length of inhalation or exhalation.
- Inducement of any tension or discomfort.
- Don't forget to measure your CP before and after any breathing exercises. And remember that measurement of CP

after regular exercise requires you to wait for some time until your breathing stabilizes to its normal level.

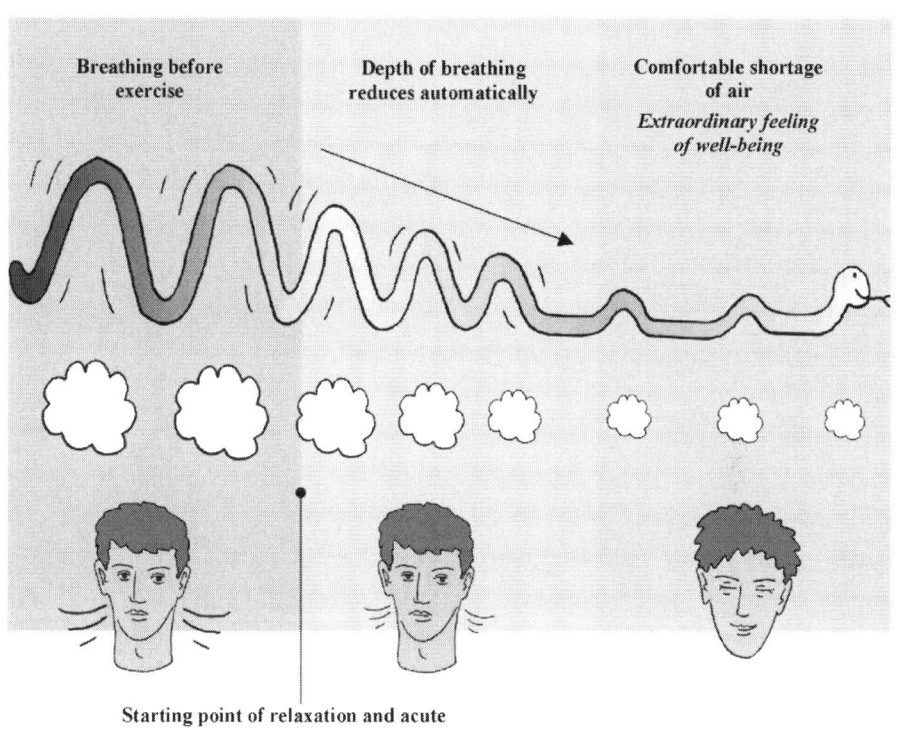

Breathing before exercise

Depth of breathing reduces automatically

Comfortable shortage of air
Extraordinary feeling of well-being

Starting point of relaxation and acute awareness and sensitivity to breathing

Part 3: Buteyko Breathing Exercises by Andrey Novozhilov, MD

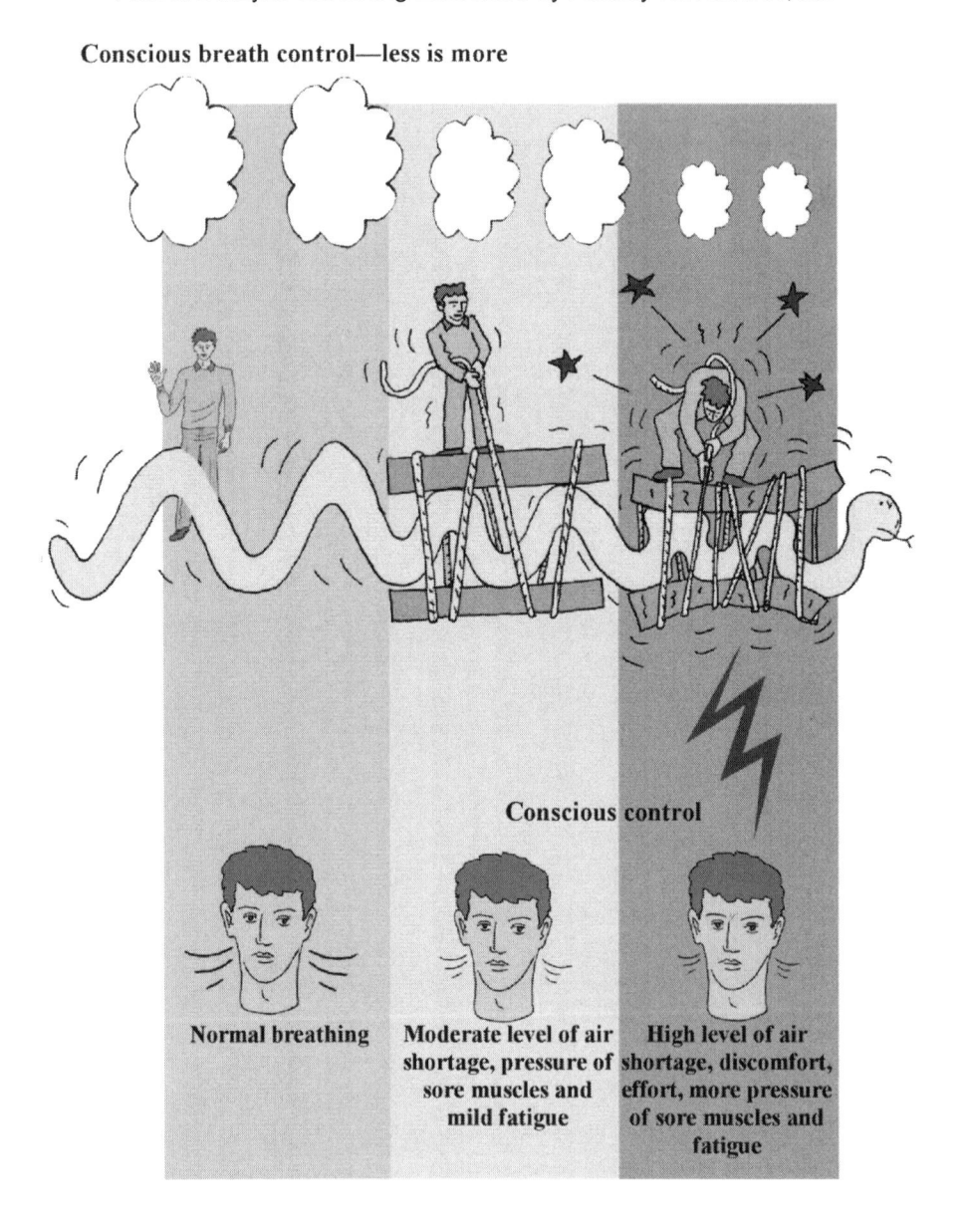

Conscious breath control—less is more

Conscious control

Normal breathing | Moderate level of air shortage, pressure of sore muscles and mild fatigue | High level of air shortage, discomfort, effort, more pressure of sore muscles and fatigue

Exercise # 2: Holding your breath

As explained previously, some people with low level of CO_2 have difficulty with Exercise # 1. If this is the case, you should try Exercises # 2, 3 or 4.

Exercise # 2 is designed to reduce the volume of breathing and increase the level of CO2 by creating a feeling of comfortable air shortage. This is achieved through willpower exerting pressure on the breathing process to create a feeling of hunger for air. This is a different feeling to that experienced in Exercise # 1, where breathing is reduced through relaxation and imagining a reduction of airflow. It does not involve willpower.

For this exercise, breathe out normally. At the end of the exhalation, hold your nose with your thumb and index finger. Try not to exhale with force, as this will result in immediate discomfort.

Continue to hold your breath until you feel a slight but comfortable feeling of air shortage.

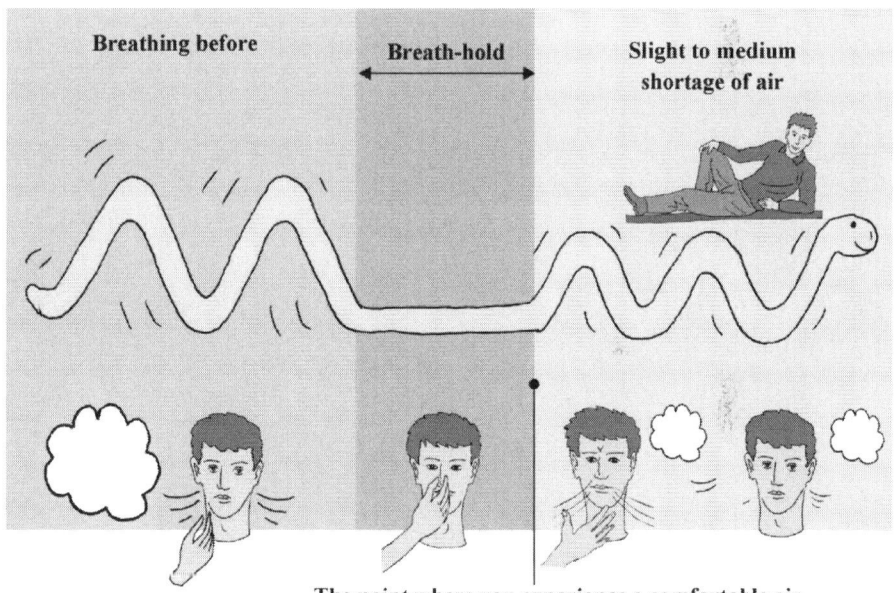

Breathing before — **Breath-hold** — **Slight to medium shortage of air**

The point where you experience a comfortable air shortage and release your nose to breath again

When you resume breathing, sustain this feeling for as long as you can.

Once you start breathing again, try to maintain a comfortable feeling of air shortage with your breathing muscles relaxed. If you try too hard to create an air shortage, this will disrupt your breathing pattern and may cause you to take deep inhalations, thus causing hyperventilation. It may help to pinch your nose during this exercise, as it is common—especially for beginners—to inhale up to 5 to 30 percent of the total volume of the lungs without being aware of it.

Possible Mistakes:
- Holding your breath for too long, resulting in an excessive shortage of air.
- Breathing pattern changed too much, as a result of excessive shortage of air.
- Any tension or discomfort during the exercise.

Exercise # 3: Holding Your Breath During Physical Exercise

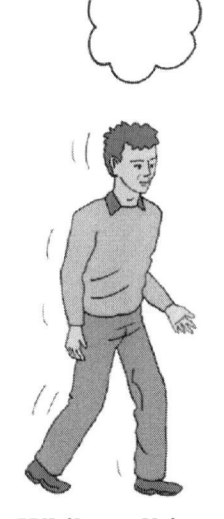

While walking

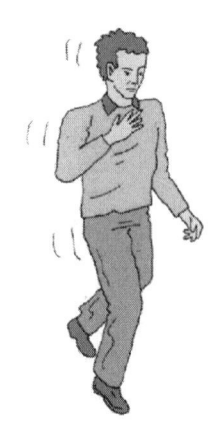

Start holding your breath after a normal exhalation by pinching your nose.

BREATHE TO HEAL

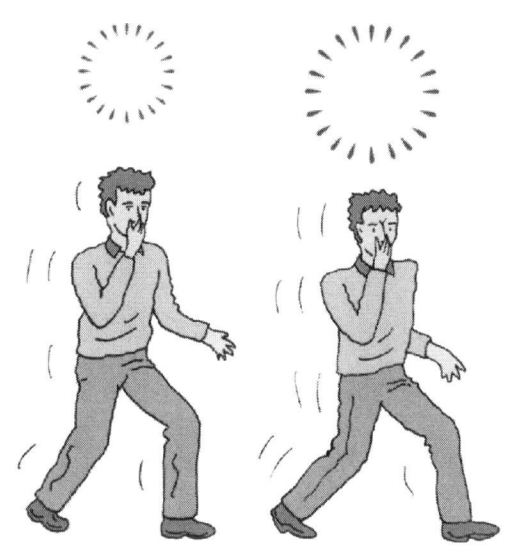

Keep walking, while experiencing an ever-increasing shortage of air from slight, to medium...

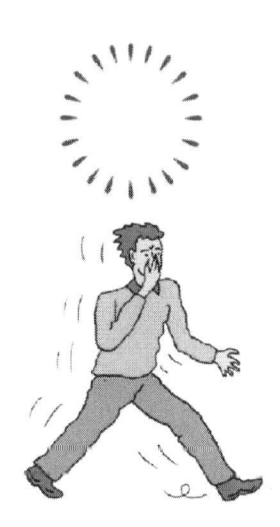

...to strong at the end. You can start to run in order to increase the air shortage even more.

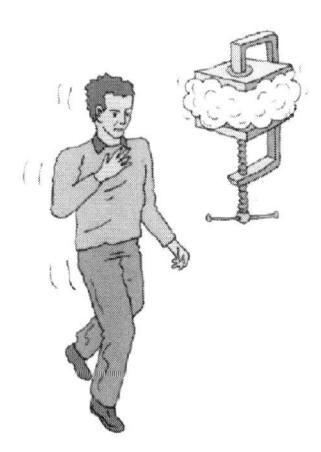

Start breathing again, before the air shortage becomes extreme. Maintain slight-to-medium air shortage for a short period.

Part 3: Buteyko Breathing Exercises by Andrey Novozhilov, MD

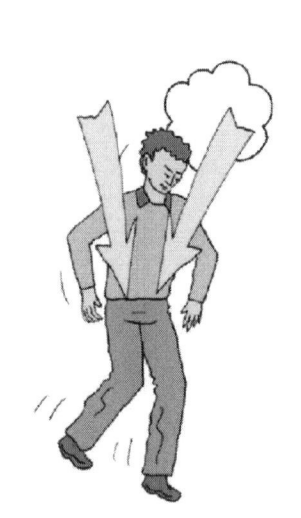

Continue walking or jogging and relax your breathing as quickly as you can by relaxing breathing muscles.

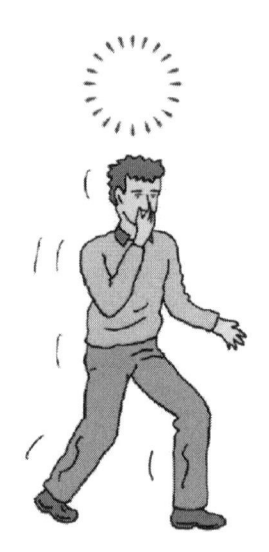

As soon as you have calmed down your breathing, you can start again.

Follow the same pattern while doing almost any type of exercise. Remember, when you resume breathing, only maintain a slight-to-medium air shortage for a short period, and calm your breathing through relaxation of breathing and other muscles.

Possible Mistakes
- Holding your breath for too long, followed by a deep breath.
- Not being able to hold your breath at all, due to extreme physical exercise.
- Maintaining air shortage for too long after you have held your breath.

Exercise # 4: Many short breath-holds throughout the day

This exercise is very useful for people who do not have the time during their workday to devote extended periods of time to other breathing exercises. With this exercise, it is possible to fit in many short breath-holds at different times throughout the day, without much disruption of your work schedule. Hold your breath to create a slight air shortage. Hold this breath for 1, 2, or 3 seconds or up to a half the length of the Control Pause, carefully avoiding any feelings of discomfort. Then, breathe normally for a while. This should be done between 100 and 500 times a day.

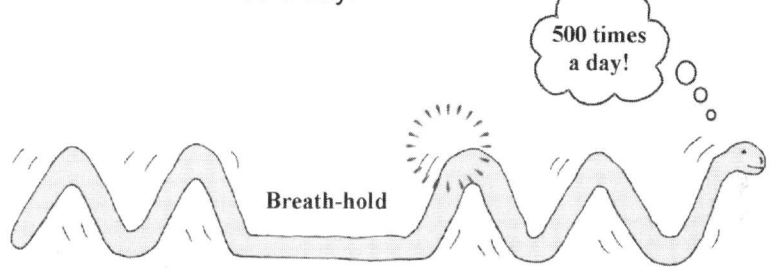

Many breath-holds during the day:
- At work—useful to combat stress
- Going to work
- When you wake up
- When you return from work
- At the cinema

Possible Mistakes:
- Air shortage becomes too big, followed by a deep breath.
- The breathing pattern changes too much, as a result of excessive air shortage.
- General tension or discomfort during exercise.

Important rules for all Buteyko breathing exercises
The greater the level of muscle activity, the more intensely you can push the feeling of air shortage.

If you are sitting still while doing the breathing exercises, the feeling of air shortage should only be very mild.

If you are exercising vigorously while doing the breathing exercises, you can push yourself to experience a stronger shortage of air.

For example, while walking, running or jumping, you can tolerate a higher level of air shortage, because your muscle activity is high. The combination of vigorous exercise and a strong feeling of air shortage produce a very high CO2 level.

When you resume breathing after holding your breath during vigorous exercise, you should keep moving while you normalize your breathing.

This breathing exercise should be repeated several times during physical exertions. The main advantage of breath holding during physical activity is that the level of CO2 increases at a substantially greater rate than it would if you were holding your breath while sitting down.

This exercise does not train us to breathe correctly. It rapidly raises the CO2 level to alleviate symptoms, but the effect is only temporary. Shortly after you stop doing the exercise, your CP will drop to where it was before. If you frequently repeat the exercise, your CP will seem to become longer, but it will not permanently raise the CO2 level until your Positive Maximum Pause has reached 40 seconds. This threshold marks the point where physiological changes enable deep breathing to be reversed permanently. You should, therefore, continue breathing exercises until this level is reached.

Caution:
As long as the Positive Maximum Pause remains between 5 and 15 seconds, this exercise should be avoided or only performed with extreme caution. Since breathing is very unstable at such low CPs, an asthma attack can be triggered by a single deep breath after a breath-hold. If it still seems sensible to work with this exercise, it should be done cautiously, slowly and with slow movements. To avoid an asthma attack, it is important not to take any deep breaths after resuming breathing.

Emergency Exercises to Combat Asthma Attack

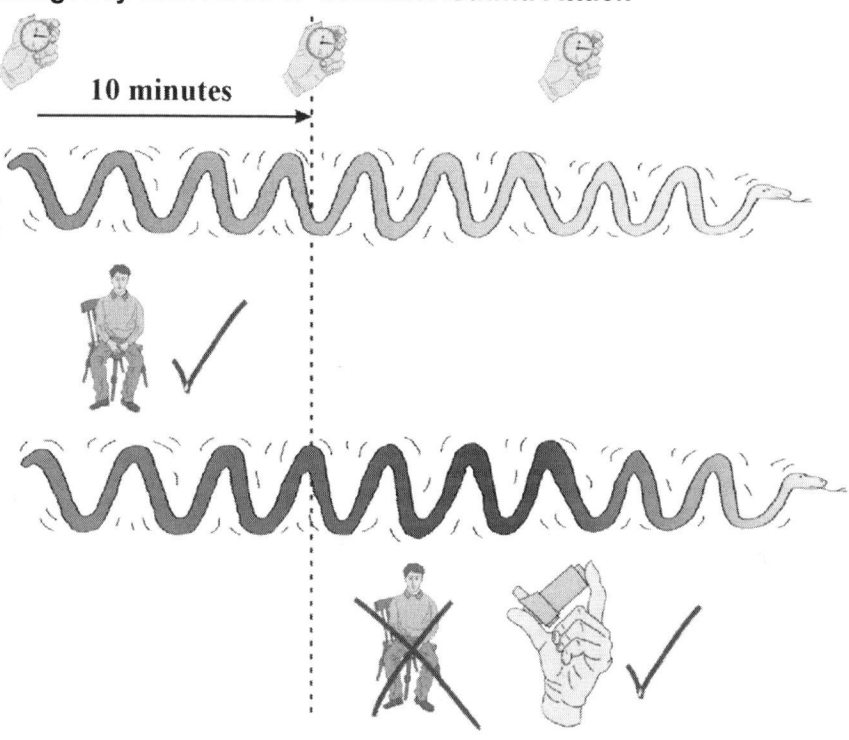

These exercises can be performed during the first stages of an asthma attack. If the attack has lasted for more than 10 minutes, it is dangerous and much more difficult to control with exercises. In this case, it is necessary to take your medication immediately.

Emergency exercise 1 – Many small breath-holds
Do many small breath-holds lasting just one or two seconds each. Space your breath-holds about one minute apart to relax and calm your breathing before taking another breath-hold.

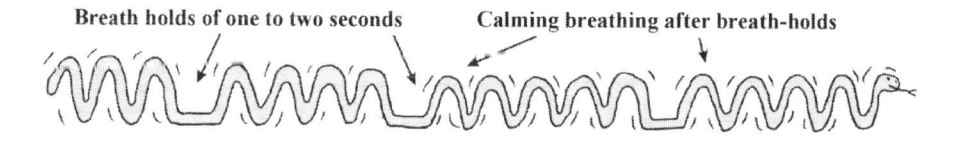

Possible Problems

The most important point to remember is that if the breath-hold is too long, the following inhalation may be too deep, resulting in an increase in the severity of the attack.

Doing breath-holds too frequently. You need to space your breath-holds far enough apart to allow your breathing to calm down before holding your breath again.

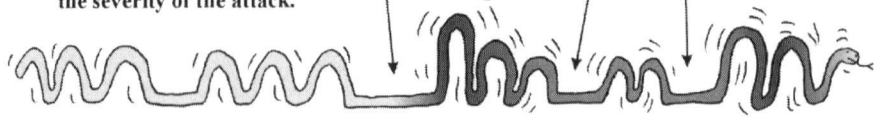

Emergency exercise 2 - Relaxation instead of exhalation

It is common to have difficulty in exhalation during an asthma attack. To help breathe out, especially during the early stages of an attack, you should do the following:

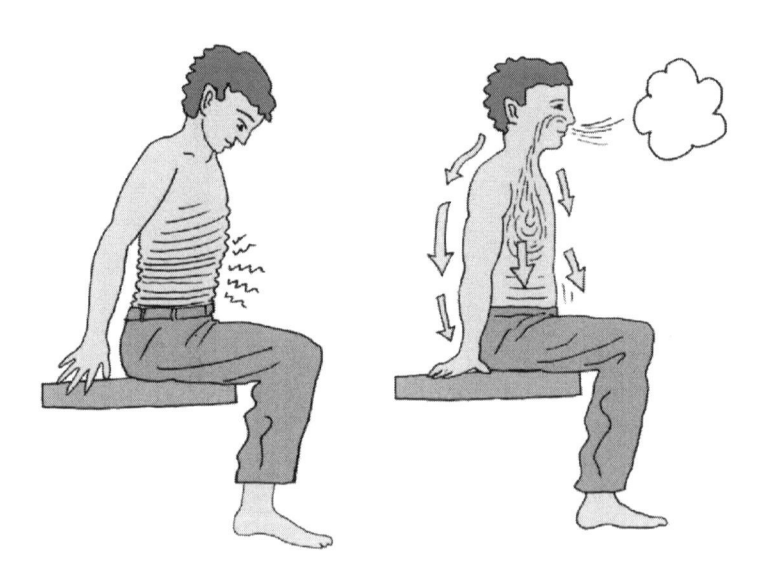

Breathe in and stop breathing for half a second. (It is not necessary to hold your breath any longer). Relax the muscles of the upper part of your stomach (above the navel) so that you breathe out naturally without any effort. Do not force your breathing. Let your relaxed muscles play the main role in the exhalation process.

Possible Mistakes:

- If the air shortage is too great, the respiratory muscles will not be able to relax.

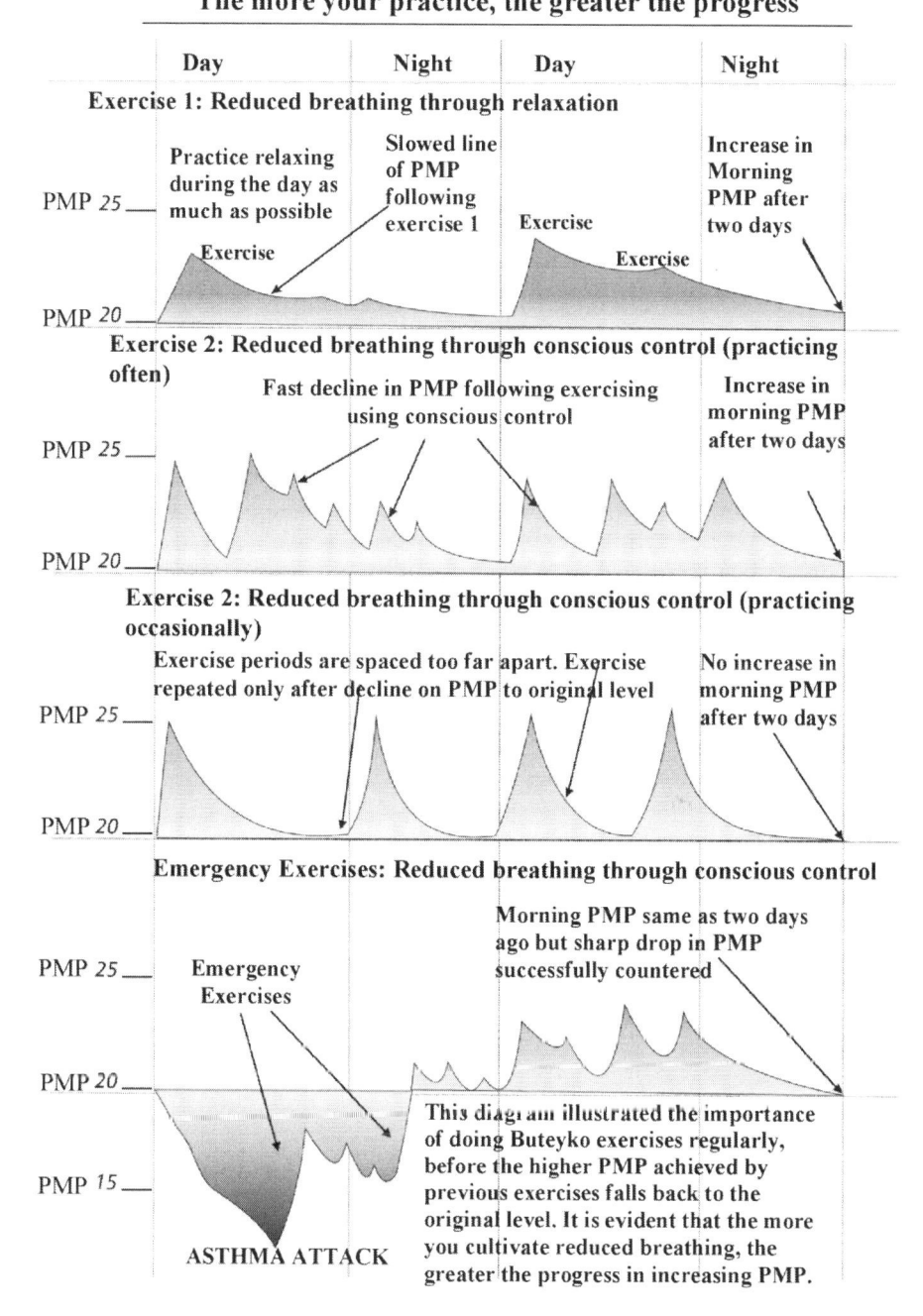

The more your practice, the greater the progress

| Day | Night | Day | Night |

Exercise 1: Reduced breathing through relaxation

PMP 25 — Practice relaxing during the day as much as possible. Slowed line of PMP following exercise 1. Exercise. Increase in Morning PMP after two days.
Exercise
PMP 20 —

Exercise 2: Reduced breathing through conscious control (practicing often)

Fast decline in PMP following exercising using conscious control. Increase in morning PMP after two days.
PMP 25 —
PMP 20 —

Exercise 2: Reduced breathing through conscious control (practicing occasionally)

Exercise periods are spaced too far apart. Exercise repeated only after decline on PMP to original level. No increase in morning PMP after two days.
PMP 25 —
PMP 20 —

Emergency Exercises: Reduced breathing through conscious control

Morning PMP same as two days ago but sharp drop in PMP successfully countered.
PMP 25 — Emergency Exercises
PMP 20 —
PMP 15 — ASTHMA ATTACK

This diagram illustrated the importance of doing Buteyko exercises regularly, before the higher PMP achieved by previous exercises falls back to the original level. It is evident that the more you cultivate reduced breathing, the greater the progress in increasing PMP.

Emergency exercise 3 - Relaxation during the exhalation

While you are exhaling, imagine your respiratory muscles relaxing, starting at the top and working down. You can tell when your respiratory muscles—especially the diaphragm—are fully relaxed by a natural pause of about half a second at the end of exhalation.

Possible Mistakes:

- Avoid holding your breath artificially at the end of exhalation. A pause at the end of exhalation should result from relaxation of the respiratory muscles, especially the diaphragm.

Exercises to Stop Symptoms:

1. Unblock your Stuffy Nose

With rhinitis or a blocked nose, you need to induce a medium or strong feeling of air shortage in order to rid yourself of the symptoms quickly. In this case, it is helpful to combine physical exercise with repeated breath holding. Stop breathing: block your nose with your fingers and start walking, running or jumping, while developing a strong feeling of air shortage. Once this feeling is strong, you must let go of your nose and resume breathing gently, taking care to avoid a deep first inhalation. Just continue walking, and try to relax and to calm down your breathing. As soon as you have calmed down, repeat the physical exercise while holding your breath again. On average, the symptoms of rhinitis will disappear within one to five minutes. This means that your nose will dry and you will be able to breathe easily. As soon as your nose is clear, there will be no need to continue with the breathing exercises because your symptoms will have disappeared.

Should the symptoms resume later, repeat the exercise until they disappear. Being able to overcome symptoms by using Buteyko exercises is very important. It builds confidence in the effectiveness of the method and provides a firm foundation for successful treatment of your asthma.

2. How to stop coughing

Coughing is a common cause of hyperventilation, as nearly everyone takes a deep breath after a cough. You can take steps to reduce hyperventilation from coughing, which should also reduce coughing itself. Coughing is both a symptom and a cause of over-breathing.

- If possible, try not to cough at all.
- Do not try to expel mucus from your bronchi with any special effort. Mucus is a protective mechanism that cannot be naturally removed until the CO2 level is sufficiently raised. When you start the Buteyko breathing exercises, the level of CO2 will increase, and the mucus will be removed without any effort. If you continue to cough, your level of CO2 will decrease, thus raising the probability of an asthma attack.
- If you do need to cough, do so without opening your mouth. Cough through your nose.

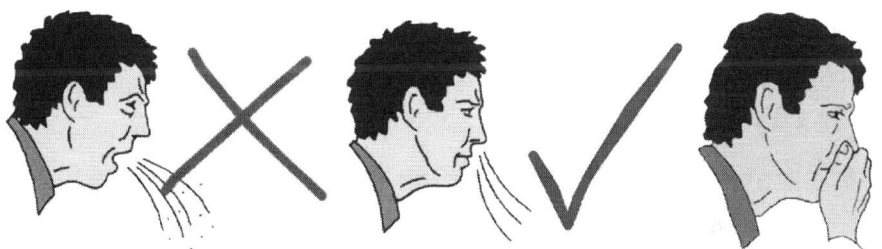

- **After each cough, hold your nose with your fingers, and hold your breath for one to three seconds to recover the loss of CO_2.**
- **When your block your nose, relax all the muscles involved with the coughing process—shoulders, thorax and upper part of the stomach.**

3. Sneezing

The same principles apply when you sneeze.

- Sneeze, stop and do a three to five-second breath-hold, and only then wipe your nose.
- Don't wipe before holding your breath because you will take a deep breath while wiping.

Part 3: Buteyko Breathing Exercises by Andrey Novozhilov, MD

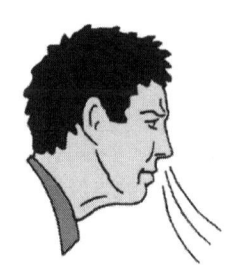

| If you have to blow, it is best to avoid trying for a thorough clearing. | You can also compensate for a loss of CO_2 by blocking your nose with your fingers and holding your breath for five seconds immediately after blowing. | It is important to wipe your nose only <u>after</u> a five-second hold. Wiping your nose before the breath-hold is likely to result in a deep inhalation while you are wiping it. |

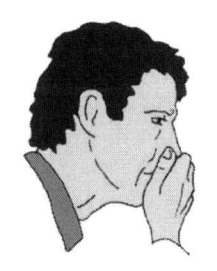

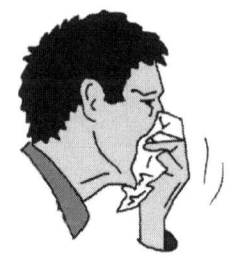

4. How to use physical exercise to control asthma symptoms:

Physical exercise is very important in helping to normalize your level of CO2. However, unless you are careful to control your breathing while exercising it may worsen your condition, especially if your Positive Maximum Pause is less than 20 seconds. If your PMP or CP is low, you should take particular care while exercising and avoid very vigorous exercise. Your aim should be to raise your PMP/CP through exercising.

The key principles to observe are as follows:

Measure your CP immediately before you start exercising.

Perform the exercise, being careful to control your breathing while exercising by:

- Maintaining a slight feeling of shortage of air all the time;
- Breathing through your nose all the time. If your PMP is greater than 20 seconds, you can breathe through your mouth briefly during strenuous phases of the exercise.

Measure your CP/PMP after exercising. If the exercise is not too strenuous, for example after a long walk or doing some housework, then you can measure your CP/PMP about 15 minutes after you have finished the activity. But if you have been exercising vigorously, then you should wait 30 minutes or even up to one or two hours before taking your CP or PMP again.

Your Control Pause or Positive Maximum Pause after the exercise must be greater than it was before you started.

If it is lower, the exercise has decreased your level of CO_2.

In this case, you need to reduce the level of your exercise to a level where you find it easier to control your breathing.

Part 4: Lifestyle Instructions

Cleansing reactions

Rehabilitation of breathing is likely to lead to so-called "cleansing reactions." These vary greatly between individuals in the type of reaction and its severity and duration. In general, the faster your progress and the more intensive your efforts to reduce breathing, the more likely cleansing reactions will occur. Around thirty percent of individuals who practice the method escape them altogether.

Cleansing reactions are usually fairly short-lived—typically two to three days—but may persist for longer. For example, mucus discharge from the nose can last for months. Every 10-second increase in the PMP is usually accompanied by one sort of cleansing reaction or another, not just mucus discharge. Often, people starting with a PMP of 10 will experience cold-like symptoms when their PMP hits around 20.

Typical reactions include

- Recurrence of the symptoms in the reverse order in which they originally manifested themselves
- Cold and flu symptoms
- Mucus discharge, sometimes spotted with blood
- Feeling poorly or just plain ill
- Headache
- Aches and pains in muscles and joints
- Nausea
- Altered sweat and urine (darker)
- Teary eyes
- Yawning
- Diarrhea

Patients often interpret these reactions as a sign that an underlying condition is worsening rather than improving. An experienced practitioner can help guide the patient through such episodes and provide encouragement and advice on how to cope with the particular symptoms involved without giving up the method. Please note that the reactions mentioned above are not comprehensive. Reactions may take many different forms.

How to prevent hyperventilation during sleep

Asthmatics will often over-breathe when they sleep, which can lead to asthma attacks at night. You can prevent hyperventilation during sleep by taking the following measures.

Measure your PMP or CP before going to sleep. Then, measure your PMP or CP again in the morning after you wake up (the Morning PMP or CP). Normally, your Positive Maximum Pause or Control Pause in the morning should be greater than it was the night before; however, it is not the same for everyone.

- If not, then you are over-breathing in your sleep. When your CP is five seconds greater after sleeping than before going to sleep, you will not have any asthma problems during the night.

- If you are already experiencing symptoms before going to sleep, your next Morning CP is likely to be lower, as breathing normally gets deeper during sleep.

- Before going to sleep, check the state of your health and consider the likelihood of a possible asthma attack during the night. If you are having severe symptoms, or you feel there is a high probability of an asthma attack during the night, it may be safer to remain awake until the threat passes or to sleep in an upright position.

- To prevent an attack, try doing breathing exercises. If this doesn't help, it may be necessary to take steroids.

- Set an alarm clock to wake yourself up every one, two or three hours, depending on the severity of your situation.

- Every time you awake, measure your CP; this will give you a good indication of the level of your health. Try to do the breathing exercises until symptoms disappear.

How to prevent hyperventilation when speaking

It is important to pay full attention to your breathing pattern at all times, whatever you are doing, even while you are speaking. If others can see you breathing while speaking, you are likely to be over-breathing. If you become aware of this, you should stop speaking immediately.

There are a number of things you can do to prevent excessive loss of CO2 while you are speaking. Do not breathe through your mouth at any time.

- Instead, shorten your sentences
- Pause
- Relax your muscles
- And, take small breaths... through the nose... in mid-sentence

Buteyko and diet

The Buteyko Method teaches you how to normalize your breathing. There is no special diet associated with the method. The Buteyko Method is about rehabilitation of breathing, not what and how much you should eat and drink.

Nevertheless, there is an important link between breathing and eating, as all food increases the depth of breathing. You can easily test this out by measuring your CP before and after a meal.

The effect of different foods and drinks varies between individuals. It helps to find out whether you are sensitive to particular types of food, and to avoid these, as they may slow down your progress.

Eventually, once you have achieved a high level of CO2 you will become more tolerant of all foods. You will then no longer need to pay so much attention to diet, provided your CP stays high. While individual response to diet varies, there are some general rules regarding the impact of diet on breathing that should guide your own habits:

- Most of us eat too much, so it may be a good idea to cut down on the amount of food you eat or miss a meal occasionally. This can make it easier to practice breath reduction over sustained periods and help you to increase your CP more quickly.
- Eat only when hungry, and only as much as you need to satisfy your hunger.
- Fresh, raw, unprocessed foods are best. Fruit and vegetables have less harmful effects on the level of CO_2 than do dairy products, meat and fish. Remember, it is not possible to normalize breathing fully just by changing your diet. It is much better to concentrate your effort on reducing breathing than in devising elaborate diets.

How to keep motivated to practice the Exercises

Many people do not persevere with the Buteyko Method for three main reasons:

- They find the exercises uncomfortable and tiring.
- Their symptoms do not improve quickly.
- They are troubled by cleansing reactions.

However, motivation can be greatly increased once you discover how to overcome symptoms by reducing your breathing.

You will also be encouraged to practice reduced breathing exercises if you discover how to make this an easy and pleasant experience.

Part 5: Use of Steroids for Asthma

Buteyko's quick and safe steroid course for asthma

> **Warning:**
> The following section is for consideration by medical professionals. This chapter is a protocol used by doctors at the Clinica Buteyko in Moscow. Do not change or adjust your medication without your doctor's approval.

With Buteyko therapy, steroids (e.g. Cortisone) are not treated simply as anti-inflammatory agents. The profound biochemical disturbances caused by chronic hyperventilation often lead to hormonal disturbances, such as insufficient cortisol production. When cortisol requirements are not met, breathing will increase, as well as the heart rate, and a general state of malaise follows. In these cases, short-term steroid supplementation is an essential adjunct to Buteyko therapy.

This chapter covers the following:

- The principles of Buteyko's short and safe steroid course
- Establishing the correct time to use steroids
- The most suitable type of steroids to use
- Protocol for applying Buteyko steroid therapy, including instructions for dose-reduction and termination of steroid therapy

Gentle Breathing

Gentle breathing enables the adrenal glands and the production of steroids to function adequately.

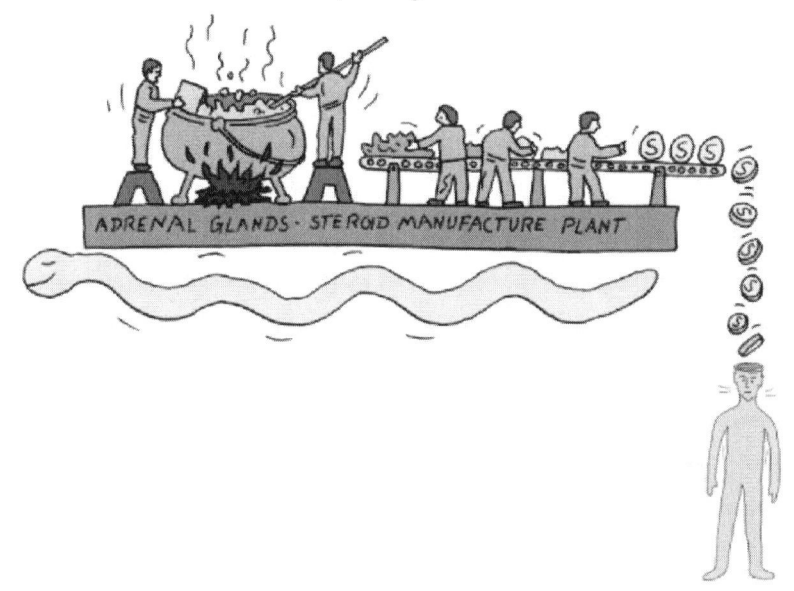

Over-breathing

Over-breathing causes biochemical disruption and impairment of adrenal gland function.

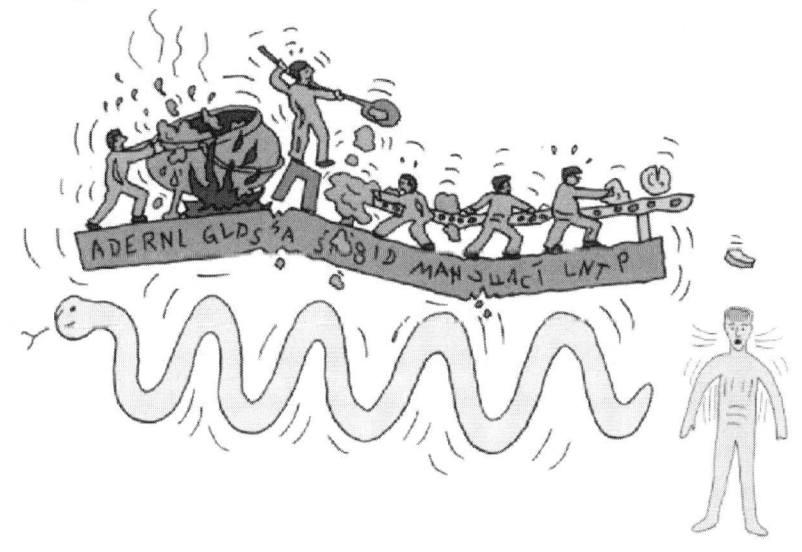

Part 5: Use of Steroids for Asthma by Andrey Novozhilov, MD

**Taking carefully measured doses of
steroids will alleviate symptoms...**

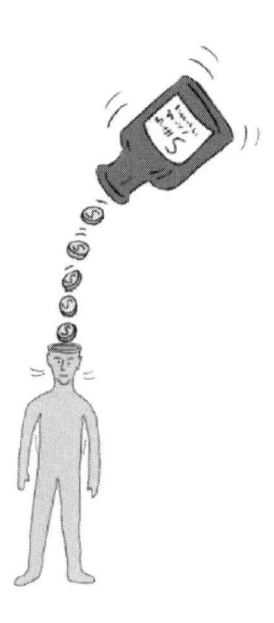

**...reduce breathing and restore proper functioning
of adrenal glands and steroid production.**

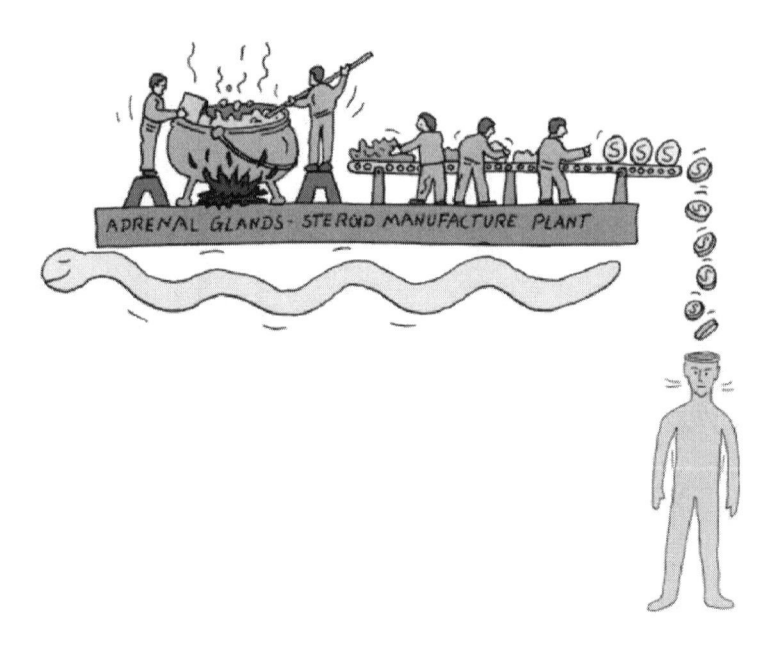

Traditional Steroid Therapy

Buteyko Short Steroid Treatment

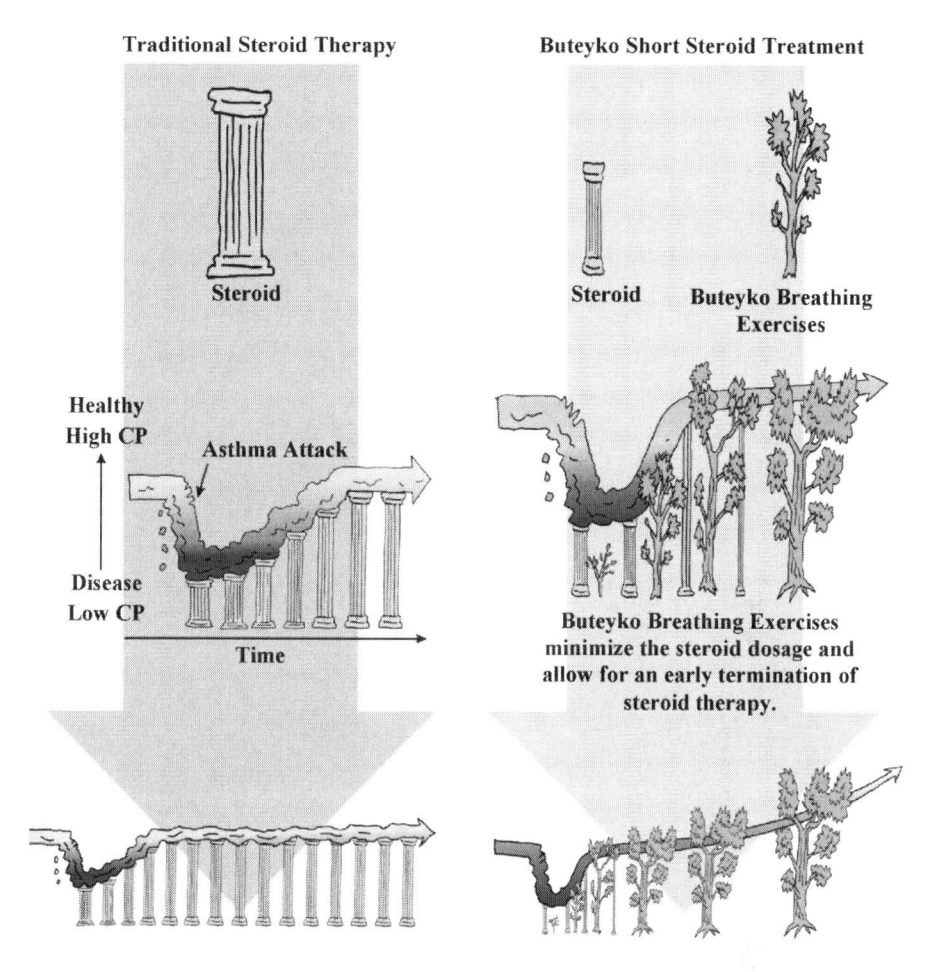

Buteyko Breathing Exercises minimize the steroid dosage and allow for an early termination of steroid therapy.

Principles

Steroids can be used briefly, safely and effectively in treating asthma. This is normally a one-time intervention, with no further application required. However, it is important to understand the principles underpinning the course and to carefully follow the procedure for deciding when to take steroids and what the appropriate dosage is.

Conventional medical management presents us with a problem. As soon as a person starts to decrease steroids, their Morning CP decreases too, either immediately or a little while later. This increases the chance of an asthma attack. A low Morning CP makes it very difficult for asthmatics to live without steroids over a long period of time once they have started to become dependent on this type of treatment. Conventional asthma management, therefore, has no way to terminate steroid therapy permanently.

The Buteyko steroid course makes it possible to wean yourself off steroids and eventually avoid asthma without the need to ever take steroids again. This is achieved by practicing Buteyko exercises diligently at the same time as small amounts of steroids are taken over a relatively short period.

The aim is to increase the Morning PMP to more than 20 seconds. Once this level is reached, you should not experience serious asthma attacks and should, therefore, be able to live without steroids. Occasionally, your PMP will drop and you may need to use steroids temporarily, but as your PMP increases, the need for steroids will gradually diminish until you no longer need steroids at all. You should be able to stop taking steroids permanently once your PMP become stable at the level of 40 seconds or more for a long period. But this goal can only be achieved if you practice breathing exercises.

The Buteyko course is safe because it requires only a low dosage of steroids. The average dose is from 0.005-0.0025 grams (one to five tablets) of Prednisolone or an equivalent, provided you start steroid therapy early enough.

It is a very short course when compared with the standard steroid therapy for asthma. If you start steroid therapy on time and with the correct dose, then the course will normally last from one to two days. If you delay starting to take steroids, it will take several more days before you can stop taking steroids; in this case, you will need to implement a dose-lowering schedule. On average, this will require about a week.

The successful application of the course is crucially dependent on doing Buteyko exercises conscientiously. This requires the patient to be strongly motivated to do the exercises and be determined to persevere, but it is well worth the effort.

What types of steroids are suitable?

Your doctor will advise you on what type of steroid to use, but you should note the following:

- It is not important what type of steroid you use. The steroid will only start working if the dose is high enough to get into your blood in sufficient quantity to affect your entire organism. Only when the steroid shortage has been fully made up will it be effective.
- The steroid dosage is more important than the type of steroid (e.g. oral, inhaled or intravenous injection).
- It is easier to control the required changes in dosage with short-acting oral steroids (tablet instead of inhaler).
- If you have other diseases such as gastritis, stomach ulcers, high blood pressure, etc. your doctor will provide you with a suitable type of steroid for your condition.

When to take steroids

There are three important indicators, which together will enable you to determine when steroids should be taken:

- **State of health**: This should be measured by your need to take a rescue inhaler such as Ventolin or its equivalent. It is important to distinguish between a "need for" and "use of" a non-steroidal rescue inhaler. It is possible for patients to ride out an asthma attack without resorting to an inhaler or to take more puffs than is necessary. It is the increased "need for" not the increased "use of" that determines whether additional steroids are required. A need for more than three puffs of a rescue inhaler in the previous 24 hours marks the beginning of asthma exacerbations and deterioration of your condition. Remember, non-steroidal medication cannot stop a seriously worsening condition.

- **Pulse**: Your "normal" pulse should be measured at rest when you are not suffering from an asthma attack. There are two main thresholds to watch out for: if your pulse exceeds 80 beats per minute (for adults), or if your pulse is 10 to 20 percent higher than your average normal pulse in the preceding 24 hours. In 80 percent of cases an increased need to take a rescue inhaler is matched by a higher pulse rate. However, in about 20 percent of cases these indicators may not be in step. For example, it is possible that your rescue inhaler requirement goes up to five to fifteen puffs per day, but your pulse initially remains close to normal. However, in such cases the pulse is likely to increase within two to three days.

- **Morning Positive Maximum Pause**: Your Morning PMP should be measured when you wake up in the morning and are still in bed. A PMP of less than 10 seconds will reinforce the need to take steroids when either of the other two indicators are flagged (i.e. the need for Ventolin more than three puffs per day, or if the pulse is raised). If your pulse is normal and you do not require 3 to 5 puffs of rescue inhaler or its equivalent per day, you should be able to increase your PMP using breathing exercises alone without taking steroids. A PMP over 10 seconds indicates a possible need to take steroids. The decision to take steroids when the PMP is over 10 seconds depends on the state of the other indicators. You should not need to take steroids if your PMP is over 20 seconds.

If you are afraid of using steroids for asthma, you can wait for all three of the above indicators to reach their critical thresholds. In this case, you will still have to use steroids, but the dose will be higher. It is, therefore, preferable to start the course earlier rather than later and to use steroids to treat asthma rather than to increase the use of a rescue inhaler (Ventolin or an equivalent) to more than three puffs per day. The following table summarizes the guidance on when to take steroids.

Example 1: Do I need to take steroids after a night of asthma attacks?

You wake up after a night of asthma attacks and are feeling unwell. You now need to decide whether you should take steroids or to increase your dose if you are already on steroids.

As previously discussed, you need to consider the three indicators that help determine what to do: You need to consider your pulse, your general state of health and your Morning PMP.

Morning PMP	Ventolin Number of puffs Needed in previous 24 hours	Pulse Above normal: Pulse exceeds 80 beats per minute (for adults) or 10-20 percent higher than average pulse of previous 24 hours.	Guidance Take steroids?
• Less than 10 seconds	• 3+ puffs	• Above Normal	• Yes
• Less than 10 seconds	• 3+ puffs	Normal	• Yes
• Less than 10 seconds	No more than 2 puffs	• Above Normal	• Yes
10+ seconds	• 3+ puffs	• Above Normal	• Yes
10+ seconds	• 3+ puffs	Normal	No
10+ seconds	No more than 2 puffs	• Above Normal	No
• Less than 10 seconds	No more than 2 puffs	Normal	No. Should be possible to increase PMP using Buteyko exercises alone
10+ seconds	No more than 2 puffs	Normal	No

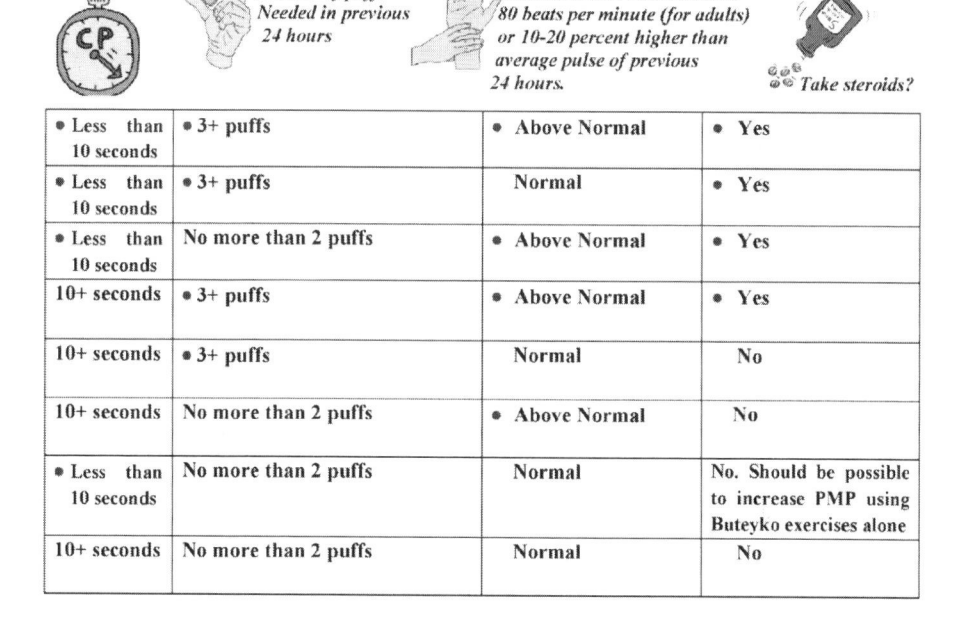

- If your pulse is 10 to 20 percent higher than your normal pulse and has not changed since the previous day, you need to take steroids or increase your dose. If you have high blood pressure, your doctor will take this into account since steroids can sometimes increase blood pressure.
- If your state of health is poor, (i.e., you required more than three puffs of a bronchodilator such as Ventolin over the

previous 24 hours), then you need to take steroids or increase your dose.

- If your Morning PMP is lower than 10 seconds but your other indicators are not so bad (e.g., your pulse is normal and you have not needed more than three puffs of Ventolin or its equivalent in the previous 24 hours) you may be able to increase your PMP with breathing exercises alone. However, if you have had a night of asthma attacks your pulse is unlikely to be normal and you will have probably taken more than three puffs of a rescue inhaler. It is likely, therefore, that you should take steroids or increase your dose.

Example 2: Will this be a low-dose, short-term course or not?

Your pulse is high, but you are not using more than one to three puffs of a rescue inhale per day. Your Morning PMP is around 15 seconds.

- It should be sufficient for you to take one to two steroid tablets during the first day while you are setting the dose. If your pulse becomes normal, your health improves sufficiently and your CP does not decrease the next morning, then you can discontinue the use of steroids immediately. If you start using steroids in time, the course will only last a day and there is no need to taper the dose off gradually.

- If you wait until your pulse becomes high and you need five to ten puffs of a rescue inhaler per day and your Morning CP drops to below 10 seconds, then you are likely to need three or more steroid tablets on the first day. The course usually lasts several days, and you will need to apply a dose-lowering schedule. This all can be avoided if you start taking the steroids in time.

Protocol for steroid therapy in the Buteyko treatment of asthma
The aim of this protocol is to find the "correct dose" of steroids for the individual on the first day. This means that the first day is dedicated to setting the dose.

1. The first day of steroid therapy for asthma

These are the rules for setting the dose:

- Measure your pulse. Increase your dose until your pulse starts to normalize. The pulse does not actually have to revert to normal immediately, but it should start to become normal.

- Consider your state of health. Increase your dose until you do not need more than one puff of a rescue inhaler (or other non-steroid inhalers) per 24-hour-period.

- Measure your Morning PMP on the day after taking the steroid. Your PMP will usually rise to over 20 seconds at the end of the dose-setting process. This might happen by the evening of the first day or by the next morning.

How to determine if the dose is correct (neither excessive nor insufficient)

If you have selected the "correct dose" you will notice the following:

- **Your pulse starts to normalize**: It need not be normal, but it must start coming down (normalizing). If you have overdosed, your pulse will slow down too quickly. If you have underdosed, your pulse does not come down within the next two days.

- **Your state of health improves**: Being in a good state of health means that while you may not have any symptoms of asthma now, you still get the occasional symptom. However, you can overcome these with Buteyko breathing exercises, or at most, one puff of a bronchodilator in 24 hours. If you overdose, you will not have any asthma symptoms at all. You can eliminate all symptoms of asthma very quickly by overdosing. Overdosing is not dangerous over short periods. However, you need to have occasional asthma symptoms in order to motivate you to work on your breathing with the Buteyko Method. If you underdose, you will need more than three puffs of a bronchodilator in 24 hours.

- **Your Morning PMP becomes greater than 20 seconds**: When the correct steroid dose has been set and administered as a result of the dose-setting process, the level of breathing will decrease automatically. A PMP of more than 20 seconds will reduce the probability of an asthma attack. If you overdose, your PMP will rise to around 30, and you will not experience any asthma symptoms. If you underdose, your PMP will drop to below 10.

You are likely to overdose if you panic at the start of an asthma attack while trying to determine your dose.

It is not dangerous to overdose on steroids for a short while. An overdose will help you to reduce your dose more quickly and make you feel much better.

A. Setting your initial dose (when you are not already on steroids) during the first day

First hour

Consider your pulse and state of health. If your pulse is between 80 and 100 and you can manage without bronchodilators, then you are not too bad. You should take only one steroid tablet immediately. If your pulse is between 100 and 120 or higher, your airways are whistling or wheezing and you need one or two puffs of bronchodilator, then your condition justifies taking two or three steroid tablets immediately.

The standard dose of a steroid tablet is 0,005 of Prednisolone or 0,004 grams of Triamcinolone or its equivalent. If you are taking the steroid in tablet form, do not swallow the tablet but suck it until it dissolves in the mouth. You should also do any Buteyko breathing exercise that does not involve physical activity. If your condition is not too bad, try to do the "relaxation instead of exhalation" exercise.

One of the features of an attack is the difficulty in breathing out. To help breathe out, especially during the early stages of an attack, perform the following:

- Breathe in and stop breathing for half a second. It is not necessary to do a breath-hold.
- Relax the muscles above your stomach so that you breathe out naturally without any effort.
- Do not force exhalation or mechanically breathe out. The exhalation process should proceed naturally through relaxation of the respiratory muscles.

If your condition is bad, try to do the exercise, "Many small breath-holds throughout the day."

- Do many small breath-holds each lasting one or two seconds.
- Allow an interval of one to two minutes between each breath-hold. During this interval, try to relax the abdominal muscles around the diaphragm.
- Remember not to hold your breath for too long; otherwise, the next breath is likely to be too deep and exacerbate the attack.

After 1–2 hours
If there is no change and you are still feeling bad with a high pulse, low CP and a need for bronchodilators, then take one more tablet.

Next 2–3 hours
Try doing breathing exercises, with particular attention to relaxing the abdominal muscles around the diaphragm. If there is still no change after two to three hours, take one more steroid tablet.

Next 3–4 hours
Continue the Buteyko breathing exercises. Remember to pay attention to relaxing the abdominal muscles around the diaphragm. If there is still no change after three to four hours, take one more tablet. Continue with the Buteyko breathing exercises.

For every subsequent 3–4 hour periods
Continue taking another tablet every three to four hours until your pulse starts to normalize and you start feeling better.

B. Correcting the dose if you are already on steroids

If you are already on steroids, you can follow the same principles as described above to optimize your dosage. An optimum dose is one which results in a good state of health. In other words, your pulse is close to normal and you can readily overcome symptoms with the Buteyko breathing exercises or with a puff of a non-steroidal inhaler no more than once in 24 hours.

You should simply adjust the amount of steroids you are taking to a level where you only occasionally have asthma symptoms. These can be readily controlled by breathing exercises. If you are already taking steroids where the dose has been set by conventional treatment for asthma, it is likely that the existing dose is more than you need to follow the Buteyko course. In this case you will need to progressively cut back your dose to a point where you can maintain a "good state of health."

1. The second day of steroid treatment for asthma
The amount of steroids taken during the first day is called the 24-hour dose. On the second day you must divide the 24-hour dose in two parts. One third of the 24-hour dose is called the daytime dose, and two thirds is called the nighttime dose.

The greater part of the 24-hour dose (two thirds of the 24-hour dose) should be taken before going to sleep at night. As it is difficult to control the volume of your breathing when you sleep, you need more steroids at night than during the day in order to decrease the volume of your breathing while you sleep.

If your daily dose is more than two tablets, then you should take this same dose for at least a few days. You should then reduce this dose gradually over the next few days.

2. Summary of the dosing process
If you have dosed yourself correctly your pulse will be normal, but you may still have the occasional symptom of asthma, which you can overcome with Buteyko breathing exercises, or at most, one puff of a non-steroidal inhaler in 24 hours.

If your health has improved to the extent that you are completely free of symptoms, and therefore, do not need to do any Buteyko breathing exercises, then you have overdosed on steroids. In this event you need to reduce your dose until the symptoms return but can still be managed quite easily with Buteyko breathing exercises. Having symptoms at this level encourages you to do the breathing exercises and will give you the experience of overcoming symptoms.

If you use a steroid but your pulse is high and you have been taking more than one to three puffs of a bronchodilator in 24 hours, then you have underdosed on steroids and need to increase the dose.

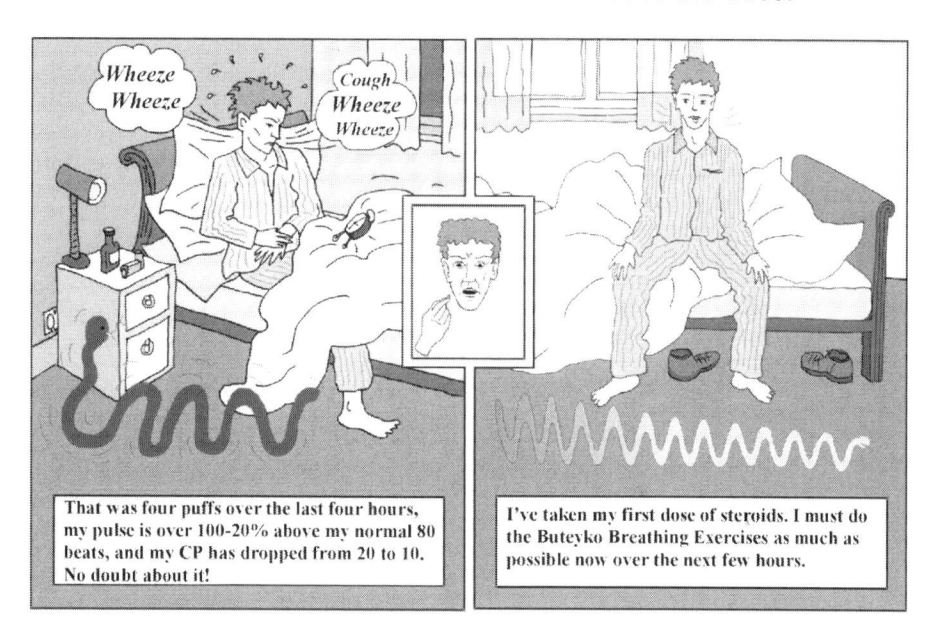

It is better to have overdosed than to have underdosed. Underdosing with steroids can be very dangerous since your asthma is then poorly controlled. With insufficient steroids it is very difficult to decrease the volume of air you breathe, even if you are trying to do Buteyko breathing exercises. This will increase the likelihood of emergency hospitalization for a severe asthma attack. You will then require much larger dosages of steroid to control your asthma.

Dose reduction and termination of steroid therapy

How long do you need to take steroids?

Theoretically, you need to take steroids until your Morning PMP becomes higher than 20 seconds. When this happens, your state of health and pulse will normalize, and you can decrease the dose and start to terminate steroid supplementation.

For how long should one stay on the same dose?

Once your asthma has normalized, you should maintain the 24-hour dose for two days, but don't forget to divide the daily dose into a daytime dose and a nighttime dose. If your health is poor during these two days and if your asthma has not stabilized, then it is necessary to increase the level of your 24-hour dose.

- If your condition is bad during the day, increase your daytime dose.
- If your condition is bad during the night, increase your nighttime dose.

When you can begin reducing your dose

If your asthma is stable for two days, then you may reduce your steroids in consultation with your doctor. If your pulse is normal and your Morning PMP is between 20 and 30 seconds, and if you are confident that your health is stable, then you can start reducing steroids earlier. If your PMP remains stable at 20 to 30 seconds, then you can start reducing steroids on the next day.

How to reduce the dose

Start by reducing your *daytime* dose first.

- The rate at which you reduce your dose depends on your state of health.
- You can reduce your daytime dose by half if you have a normal pulse and a PMP from 20 to 30 seconds.
- If in doubt, reduce the daytime dose only by a quarter.

Don't reduce your *nighttime* dose until you have completed reducing the daytime dose to zero. Only when you are no longer taking steroids during the day should you start to reduce your nighttime dose The course of steroid treatment should last from one to two days to one to two weeks, depending on the 24-hour dose and your CP.

What should you do if your condition deteriorates while reducing the steroid dosage?

Your condition will deteriorate only when your PMP or CP starts to reduce. You will have to postpone reducing steroids. You should increase your dosage again and do breathing exercises more actively until your pulse becomes normal and your PMP stabilizes at more than 20 seconds.

- If you deteriorate during the day, increase the daytime dose.
- If you deteriorate during the night, increase the nighttime dose.
- You may not need to increase the overall 24-hour dose.

Resume dose reduction when your pulse becomes normal and your Morning PMP is more than 20 seconds.

How to avoid having to resort to further steroid interventions

As long as your Morning PMP is higher than 20 seconds you will not experience any serious asthma attack. Therefore, your initial aim should be to achieve a Morning PMP of more than 20 seconds. Steroids and Buteyko breathing exercises will help you achieve this level of Morning PMP. You should not need to take steroids provided you can keep your Morning PMP above 20 seconds with the help of the Buteyko breathing exercises. However, until your Morning PMP become stable at least 40 seconds you will not have reversed asthma, as you will still be susceptible to temporary PMP drops to below 20 seconds, which are likely to be accompanied by a return of asthma attacks.

In order to reverse asthma completely and never require any further steroid therapy, you need to have a Morning PMP greater than 40 seconds for at least six months. This will require continued application of the Buteyko breathing exercises until you achieve a consistently high Morning PMP of over 40 seconds, preferably 60 seconds.

Buteyko therapy compared with traditional treatment for asthma

There are a number of shortcomings of conventional medicine:

- It does not tailor the dose to an individual's needs. There are no clear guidelines and no signs to follow for setting the dose, apart from "good health," "bad health," and "getting better."

- While conventional treatment can make the patient feel well very quickly, this usually leads to doses that are too high.

- It prescribes a *daytime-dose* that is the greater part of the *24-hour dose.* Failure to recognize the need for a higher dose while asleep (when it is more difficult to control breathing) is more likely to cause health problems at night.

- Conventional treatment tries to wean the patients off steroids gradually, irrespective of the state of health. Even when the health deteriorates, doctors continue to reduce steroids supplementation.

In contrast, the Buteyko therapy for asthma:

- Tailors the dose to an individual's needs and provides clear guidelines for setting the dose;

- Recognizes the need for higher doses at night;

- Avoids overdosing because it is short and requires a lower dose of steroids;

- Enables the patient eventually to live without having to take steroids ever again and be cured of asthma;

- But the Buteyko Method dies depend on the patient doing the breathing exercises diligently.

BREATHE TO HEAL

The quick and safe Buteyko steroid course

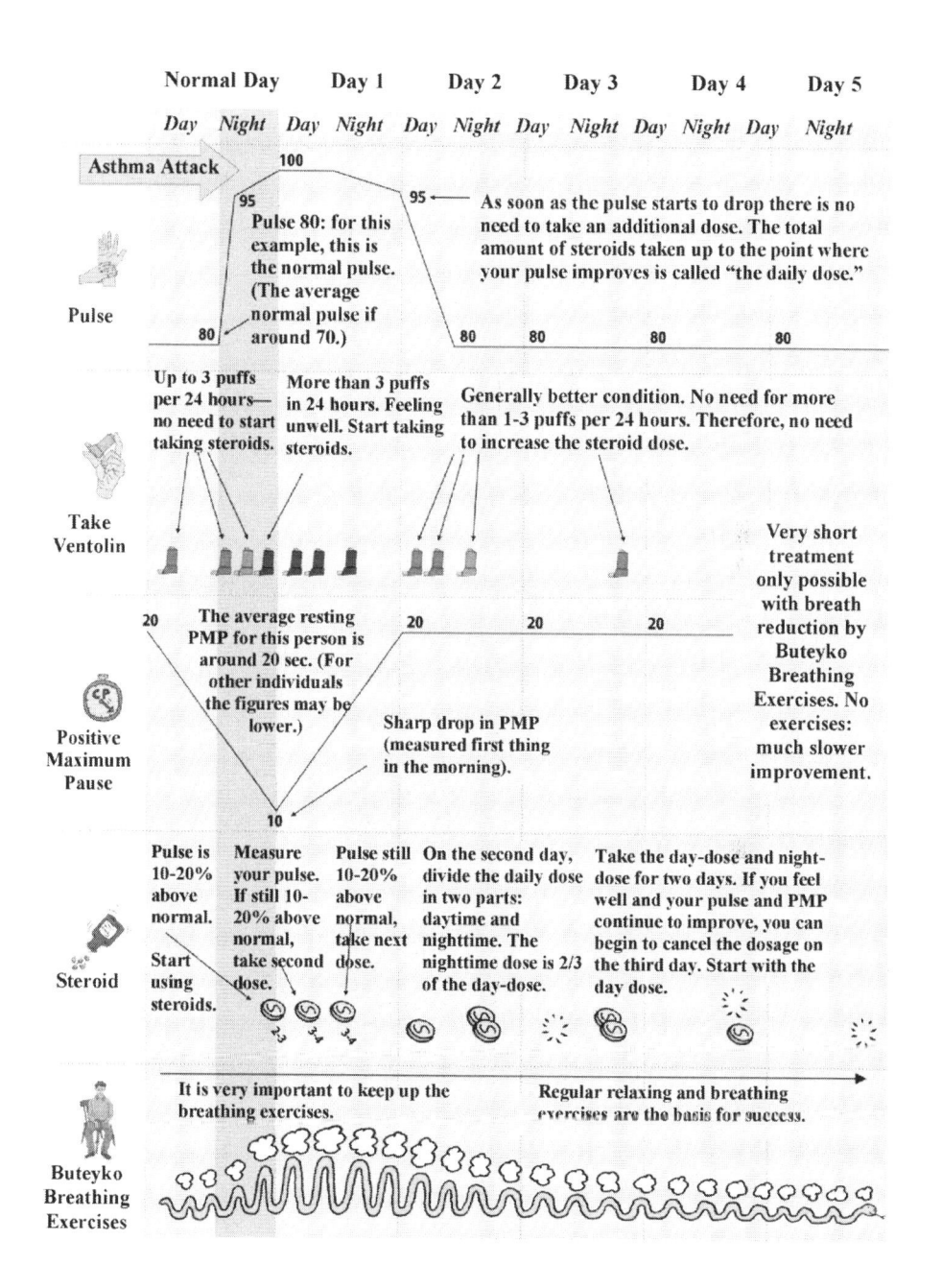

	Normal Day	Day 1	Day 2	Day 3	Day 4	Day 5
	Day Night	Day Night	Day Night	Day Night	Day Night	Day Night

Asthma Attack

Pulse

- 100
- 95 — Pulse 80: for this example, this is the normal pulse. (The average normal pulse if around 70.)
- 95 ← As soon as the pulse starts to drop there is no need to take an additional dose. The total amount of steroids taken up to the point where your pulse improves is called "the daily dose."
- 80, 80, 80, 80, 80

Take Ventolin

- Up to 3 puffs per 24 hours—no need to start taking steroids.
- More than 3 puffs in 24 hours. Feeling unwell. Start taking steroids.
- Generally better condition. No need for more than 1-3 puffs per 24 hours. Therefore, no need to increase the steroid dose.
- Very short treatment only possible with breath reduction by Buteyko Breathing Exercises. No exercises: much slower improvement.

Positive Maximum Pause

- 20
- The average resting PMP for this person is around 20 sec. (For other individuals the figures may be lower.)
- 20, 20, 20
- 10
- Sharp drop in PMP (measured first thing in the morning).

Steroid

- Pulse is 10-20% above normal. Start using steroids.
- Measure your pulse. If still 10-20% above normal, take second dose.
- Pulse still 10-20% above normal, take next dose.
- On the second day, divide the daily dose in two parts: daytime and nighttime. The nighttime dose is 2/3 of the day-dose.
- Take the day-dose and night-dose for two days. If you feel well and your pulse and PMP continue to improve, you can begin to cancel the dosage on the third day. Start with the day dose.

Buteyko Breathing Exercises

It is very important to keep up the breathing exercises.

Regular relaxing and breathing exercises are the basis for success.

141

SECTION 5: BREATHING NORMALIZATION FOR CHILDREN

By Sasha Yakovleva
Illustrations by Arash Akhgari

This section is written for parents who wish to help their children to reduce or stop asthma symptoms by applying Dr. Buteyko's approach—the Breathing Normalization Method. In this part of the book, I share my experience as a Breathing Normalization Specialist who worked with many children suffering from asthma. I apologize if some information, which you learned in the previous sections of this book, is repeated here. If so, it is presented from a specific angle of work with children. Nevertheless, all recommendations in this section are applicable not only to children but to adults as well.

Part 1: Breathing and its Measurements

Over-Breathing

According to Dr. Buteyko and Dr. Novozhilov, the trigger for asthmatic symptoms is over-breathing. Over-breathing, or hyperventilation, is dangerous for many reasons but primarily because it lowers the CO2 level in the alveoli of the lungs, which, as Dr. Buteyko stated, is the main regulator of most bodily functions. Since hyperventilation can be lethal, the human body will try to protect itself from hyperventilating in various ways, including by creating mucus, coughing, out of breath feeling and other asthmatic symptoms children often experience.

Reducing air consumption can reduce or eliminate hyperventilation. In a healthy child, the body usually accomplishes this by narrowing the airways through generating excess mucus (leading to a runny or stuffy nose) or coughing. If this tactic is not effective, then the body resorts to stronger defense mechanisms such as gasping for air, enlarging the tonsils and adenoids or creating suffocation attacks. By creating these "problems", the body is desperately trying to lessen its air exchange.

When a child learns how to breathe less (resulting in increased level of CO^2 in the lungs), hyperventilation is tamed. Then the body no longer needs to come up with compensatory mechanisms, and the symptoms described above are reduced or disappear entirely.

It usually takes between two and four months to establish healthy breathing patterns, though the positive results of better breathing become evident within the first two weeks of Breathing Normalization training. The transition from excessive breathing to healthy breathing can be time-consuming, since changing lifelong habits is never easy. But the effort is well worth it: healthy breathing patterns create a solid foundation for optimal health for the rest of the child's life.

Health cannot exist without healthy breathing. When a child's breathing becomes "normal" by Dr. Buteyko's standards (stable Positive Maximum Pause of 60 seconds or higher), he becomes disease-free. That means not having to deal with breathing difficulties, colds, ear infections, allergies, or any kind of respiratory problems. This is the best gift a parent can offer their child!

Healthy Breathing

Children with asthma mainly breathe through their mouth. Their shoulders, chest and stomach often move with every inhalation and exhalation; their breathing is audible and is often followed by wheezing. An asthmatic child can sit on a sofa watching TV and breathe as heavily as if he is running.

In marked contrast to hyperventilation, healthy breathing is unnoticeable. The ideal breath is so light and gentle that it cannot be observed. It looks as though the person is not breathing at all! His shoulders, chest and stomach barely move, his inhalations and exhalations are silent, and his mouth is closed, unless he is eating or talking.

Nasal breathing is the most important element of healthy breathing. Dr. Buteyko said that any child who breathes through his mouth instead of his nose is seriously ill, regardless of whether or not he expresses disease symptoms.

Through Breathing Normalization training, a child becomes able to breathe through his nose all the time—during studying, socializing, sleeping, talking, eating, and physical activities.

Close Your Mouth

Mouth breathing is often responsible for the flu, as well as many other viral infections, which for an asthmatic child are very dangerous. When you breathe through your mouth, you are basically creating a microbe highway from the outside environment directly into your air passages. In addition, the air itself is often over-cooled and unprepared for consumption. A healthy body temperature is 97.88 degrees Fahrenheit. Air any cooler than that contributes to a gradual breakdown of the immune system and can lead to respiratory problems.

"Mouth breathing," says Dr. Novozhilov, "is often the sole reason for chronic tonsillitis and enlarged adenoids in children, which causes frequent colds and bronchitis, and eventually ends with surgical intervention." Of course, on top of it all, it also triggers asthma.

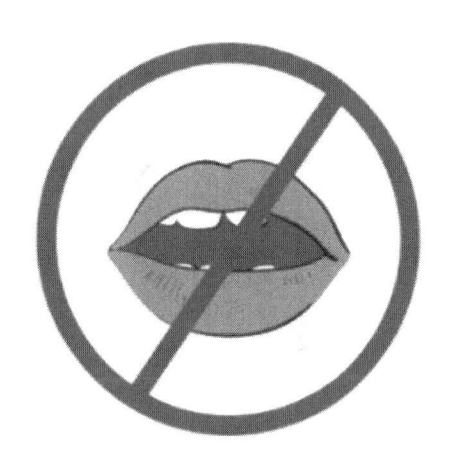

Nasal breathing is the simple solution, one that you or your child can start practicing right away, and one that Dr. Novozhilov says "is quite effective in shielding the body against viruses, such as a seasonal flu." A flu virus spreads through infected droplets that fly off a sick person when he coughs, sneezes or even speaks. These droplets can travel up to fifty feet from their source, and are so tiny that they can penetrate even the space between the fibers of a paper or cloth mask. Thus, during a flu pandemic, it is nearly impossible to avoid infected areas and to prevent the virus from finding its way into your body.

Fortunately, the way the virus enters your body can make all the difference. The majority of viruses cannot survive on the mucus membrane of the nose. The microbes in this membrane create a hostile environment for the virus. When breathing through your nose, you are sterilizing the air entering your body, creating a shield against disease. Nasal breathing warms the air, moistens it, and conditions it for perfect consumption.

Healthy nasal breathing is the main treatment for asthma (and many other health issues) and a way to prevent the problem in the first place. Healthy breathing is simple, although it takes time and energy for any person, adult or child, to unlearn a lifetime's worth of unhealthy breathing habits. Parents need to be patient when teaching their child how to breathe lightly and through the nose only.

While it may be easy for parents to breathe through their noses, it could be extremely arduous for their asthmatic child. This is one of the reasons it is recommended that parents work with a Breathing Normalization Specialist who can make this healing journey less difficult.

Sometimes it is almost impossible for a child to breathe through his nose at all, especially at night. In this case, the parent faces a dilemma: should my child breathe through his mouth or should I use medication to open his airways? In this instance, the use of medication is recommended to open the air passages and make it possible for the child to do the breathing exercises. As the child's treatment progresses, medication will not be needed.

It is also important to realize that even though nasal breathing greatly reduces hyperventilation, it does not always stop it. A child who breathes through his nose can still hyperventilate to some degree. The best sign that hyperventilation is eliminated is indicated by greatly improved breathing measurements.

Why does my child hyperventilate?
Many parents assume that healthy breathing is supposed to come naturally. They are puzzled about why their child over-breathes.

Healthy or natural breathing is the result of a natural lifestyle. Most modern children don't follow a natural lifestyle, so their breathing patterns are disturbed. Unnatural breathing patterns can be corrected through lifestyle changes in combination with breathing exercises.

One of the main causes of hyperventilation in children is the intake of antibiotics. Antibiotics do not discriminate; once they enter the body, they not only attack illness-producing bacteria, but also the beneficial bacteria that live in many places throughout the body, most especially in the upper airways and the intestinal tract. When these populations of beneficial bacteria are depleted, the body cannot perform many functions properly, breathing among them.

In the United States, antibiotics are often prescribed to children when they have a common flu, cold or infection. Sometimes, doctors prescribe them as a precaution, worrying that without them a child's ailment might get worse. Considering the harmful effects of antibiotics on breathing and the body in general, doctors at Clinica Buteyko Moscow recommend that parents and doctors practice extreme caution in their application. Antibiotics are useful for life-threatening situations, but it is better to avoid them if a child is only mildly ill. And in every case, healthy breathing is the best protection from any respiratory issues, as well as many other health problems.

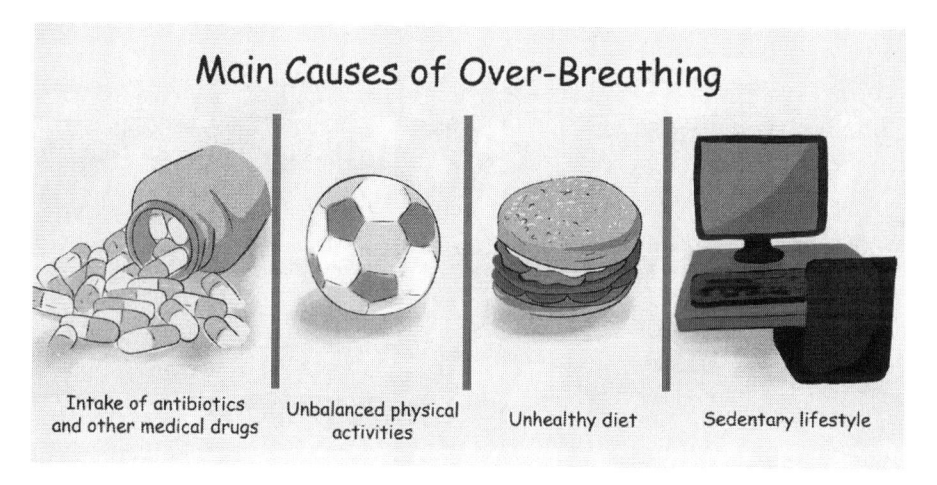

Main Causes of Over-Breathing

| Intake of antibiotics and other medical drugs | Unbalanced physical activities | Unhealthy diet | Sedentary lifestyle |

Other common causes of hyperventilation include an imbalance of physical activities, improper diet and the stresses of everyday life. These topics are covered in detail in the next part of this section.

Breathing Measurements:
In order to understand the state of your child's health and track his progress through his healing process, you need to learn how to measure his breathing.

There are two types of breathing measurements: **Control Pause** and **Positive Maximum Pause.** Both are indicators of the CO2 level in the alveoli of the lungs. A certain minimal level of CO2 in the lungs is essential for good health. A low *Control Pause* or *a low Positive Maximum Pause* shows that the carbon dioxide level in the lungs is insufficient. Higher breathing measurement numbers indicate a higher level of carbon dioxide in the lungs, and therefore, equates with better health. The goal of Breathing Normalization training is to reestablish the normal carbon dioxide level. My experience has shown that some children are not able to achieve this level. However, moving closer to it (to any degree!) proportionally improves the child's state of health. Children who are able to reach a level above normal become extremely healthy—practically disease-free.

For most people the idea of accumulating carbon dioxide seems counterintuitive. We all know that oxygen is essential for life, and we are taught to think of CO2 as a waste product. Dr. Buteyko pointed out that oxygen cannot be delivered to various organs of the body if the CO2 level in the lungs is low. Carbon dioxide regulates pH, which regulates oxygen delivery! Unless there is sufficient carbon dioxide in the bloodstream, oxygen molecules "stick" to the red blood cells and cannot be released to the cells that need them. Carbon dioxide is not a nutrient, the way oxygen is; it is more like a key that, when fitted into the chemical lock, releases oxygen. To learn more about this scientific principle, I suggest reading about the *Bohr effect*.

Breathing measurements are also indicative of the oxygenation of a child's whole body. As your child's Control Pause rises, you may notice that he will begin to look healthier. The typical pale look will be replaced with rosy cheeks. He will become more energetic, but also calmer and better able to focus.

How to take breathing measurements
Measuring one's breathing is not a contest to see how long a person can hold his breath! Attempting to hold one's breath as long as possible causes stress, which, in turn, causes hyperventilation. This, of course, is the opposite of what you are trying to achieve.

1. Control Pause:

The Control Pause is the length of time a person can comfortably go without taking a breath following a light exhalation. The ability to sense the point at which "comfort" turns into discomfort can take adults weeks of practice to develop. So it's unrealistic to expect a child to be able to do this perfectly. The goal is to sense the moment at which the body wants to inhale. This is quite a subtle sensation, so the best way to approach it is to periodically remind the child of the instructions and ask him if he feels he understands them.

Instructions:

Ask the child to sit in a chair with a hard surface. His mouth has to remain closed throughout the whole measurement. Have him inhale and exhale a few times, paying attention to his breathing. Then, ask him to block his nose <u>after exhaling</u> and stop breathing. When he feels the need to breathe again, he should gently inhale through his nose. This measurement requires very little effort, almost none.

2. Positive Maximum Pause:

Description:

Positive Maximum Pause is longer than Control Pause and is a bit more difficult to measure. To follow a Positive Maximum Pause measurement a person should still be able to inhale only through his nose, though the inhalation may be slightly forced. With the Positive Maximum Pause, there is always a risk of holding the breath so long that the following inhalation is through the mouth instead of the nose. Avoid this mistake at all costs.

Instructions:

Have the child sit on a chair with a hard surface. His mouth has to remain closed throughout the whole measurement. Ask him to inhale and exhale a few times, paying attention to his breathing. Then, ask him to block his nose <u>after exhalation</u> and pause his breathing. When he feels the need to breathe again, he should *wait a little longer*, and then open his nose and inhale through his nose. This measurement requires a slight effort.

- For very young children, I suggest introducing only the Control Pause. The Positive Maximum Pause may be too confusing for them.
- For older children, I suggest practicing both pauses a few times, so they understand the difference between them. After that, keep it simple by measuring the Control Pause only.

Realistically, when you ask your child to measure his Control Pause, he will be measuring something in between his Control and Positive Maximum pauses. Don't worry—this is to be expected. You need a reference point, which we will call "Control Pause," even if it is a bit higher than an actual Control Pause. A possible range of 2 to 4 seconds is acceptable, and not essential at the beginning of a breathing training. What is important is whether the Control Pause increases after doing breathing exercises, as well as over the course of weeks, months and years.

You will need to measure your child's Control Pause (and hopefully your own!) on a daily basis to measure your child's breathing. At the beginning of the training, I suggest measuring the Positive Maximum Pause only occasionally, in order to evaluate your own or your child's state of health more precisely.

Some children are very attached to the idea of achieving a high Control Pause. Of course, attaining high numbers is a good motivator, but it can also lead to cheating. Some children push too hard, inhale slightly through their mouth, or come up with other creative tricks. I remember an eight-year-old boy who tried to please his mother by demonstrating a high Control Pause. According to his breathing measurements, his Control Pause was 7 minutes! Astonishingly, his mother believed him, and even complained to me that, despite his astronomical Control Pause, the boy was still suffering from rhinitis and enlarged adenoids. When I measured his real Control Pause, it was only 12 seconds. Please watch your child's breathing measurements closely!

When to take breathing measurements

- Measure your child's Control Pause first thing every morning. Have him sit, ask him to block his nose and take the measurement. The Morning Control Pause is the most important record of the child's healing journey, so record it every day. You will also need to measure your child's Control Pause before and after each session of breathing exercises.

- For <u>a session without movement</u>, measure the Control Pause before the session and 3 to 5 minutes after the session. I recommend using this brief interlude after the session for relaxation.

- For <u>a session in motion</u>, measure the Control Pause before the session, and then 15, 30, 45 or 60 minutes after it. The number of minutes between the end of the session and when the post-session Control Pause is taken depends on the intensity of the session. If the session was not intense, the post-session Control Pause can be measured after 15 minutes. If it was very intense, wait a full hour before measuring the Control Pause. As a general rule, the post-session Control Pause should be taken once the breathing calms down again, which can take from 15 to 60 minutes after finishing a physical activity.

If you are not sure which length of time to use, try measuring the Control Pause four times—15, 30, 45 and 60 minutes after a session in motion—on successive days, using the same breathing exercise. Use the highest number. This experiment will allow you to determine the best length of time to wait before measuring your post-session Control Pause.

Important: If breathing exercises are done correctly, the post-session Control Pause should be higher than the one before it. A session without movement should generate a Control Pause increase of at least 2 seconds. A session in motion usually generates an increase of at least 5 seconds. If the post-session Control Pause is lower than pre-session one, then the breathing exercises were done incorrectly and produced a negative effect. Always remember to measure both before and after Control Pauses when doing breathing exercises. You will need these measurements to evaluate how effective the application of exercises is.

How to record breathing measurements

Record your child's breathing measurements (as well as your own) in a logbook or journal. The *Breathing Log Book* is an important tool; you will find page samples at the end of this section. Please use it to keep track of breathing improvement progress.

Here is a sample day:

Tuesday, October 22nd Morning Control Pause—13 seconds.
1st session at 6.30 am: 30 min of seated breath holds. Control Pause before: 15 sec; Control Pause after: 18 seconds.
2nd session at 4 pm: 30 min on a treadmill with breath holds. Control Pause before: 14 seconds; Control Pause after: 19 seconds.
3rd session at 8.30 pm: 30 min (10 min—airplane and other games; in bed—humming, breathing through one nostril and relaxation). Control Pause before: 18 seconds; Control Pause after: 20 seconds.

It is important to track progress over the course of months, both to confirm that what you are doing is actually working and to motivate you to continue the healing process.

How to read breathing measurements

If a child's (or adult's, for that matter) Control Pause is less than 10 seconds, then that person is very ill. For asthmatic children, this is often the case, and it should serve as a definite indicator that the child should not be forced to follow the typical hyperactive schedule that most children have today.

Following is a chart created by Dr. Buteyko that shows, in detail, the significance of breathing measurements. Breathing measurements are interpreted in a very similar way for both children and adults.

The body conditions and criteria of lung ventilation according to Dr. Buteyko:

HEALTH STATUS	BREATHING	DEGREE OF ABNORMA-LITY	CO2 in ALVEOLI % (millimeters of mercury)		POSITIVE MAXIMUM PAUSE (seconds)	PULSE (beats per minute)
Super Endurance and Longevity	Gentle Breathing	VII	Special Conditions			
		VI				
		V	7.5	53.5	180	48
		IV	7.4	52.8	150	50
		III	7.3	52	120	52
		II	7.1	50.6	100	55
		I	6.8	48.5	80	57
The Norm (Optimal Health)			6.5	46.3	60	60
Disease	Excessive Breathing	I	6	42.8	50	65
		II	5.5	39.2	40	70
		III	5	35.7	30	75
		IV	4.5	32.1	20	80
		V	4	28.5	10	90
		VII	3.5	25	5	100
DEATH						

The norm:

According to Dr. Buteyko, a truly healthy person has a Positive Maximum Pause of 60 seconds, and a Control Pause of more than 30 seconds. This means that for this child, it is not challenging to go without air for one minute, and easy to do it for half a minute. This child does not have any negative symptoms, and his immune system protects him from respiratory problems, as well as from many serious health issues, including asthma and allergies. This state of 'perfect health' does not occur when PMP reaches 60 seconds just a few times. A child belongs to this category only when his PMP is 60 seconds or higher <u>all the time</u>—day and night, especially in the morning—for at least six months.

Today, it is extremely rare to meet a child, who belongs to this category. Children suffering from mucus, coughing, wheezing, and other asthmatic symptoms are far away from this level. If a child's PMP and CP are below the norm, it means that his health is compromised.

1st Level of Hyperventilation:

If a child's PMP is consistently between 40 and 60 seconds, he or she is very healthy. At this point, a child normally does not have any asthmatic symptoms, although his immune system can be still not strong enough to completely protect him or her from disease. If a child catches flu, for example, it can lower his PMP and CP resulting re-occurrence of asthma symptoms; however, they will be controllable.

2nd Level of Hyperventilation:

If your child's PMP is in the range of 25 and 40 seconds, he belongs to the category of the semi-healthy. You might actually think of him as a healthy person, and if so, this means he has health issues you are not aware of or ones you consider normal. These issues (for example, runny nose or allergies) are common, but not normal. These symptoms will go away if you improve your child's breathing. If his PMP is closer to 25 seconds, he might still have symptoms of various diseases.

3rd Level of Hyperventilation:

If your child's PMP is between 10 and 25 seconds, he or she is not healthy. When he breathes in, he is breathing in several times more air than his body needs. This creates a negative impact on all of his body's systems and throws many functions out of balance. He likely has active asthma symptoms and his energy level is low, though he could be hyperactive at the same time. It is also possible that your child has difficulties to stay focused.

4th Level of Hyperventilation:

Dr. Buteyko stated that if someone's PMP is below 10 seconds, he is severely ill, whether they are a child or adult, whether or not they have symptoms, and whether or not they are aware of it. A person from this category is emotionally vulnerable; he may have a poor memory, difficulty focusing, low self-esteem, and chronic fatigue. A child might have very strong asthma symptoms and most likely is on strong medication. It is critical for such a child to improve his or her breathing. If not, the problem will become increasingly difficult to correct.

5th Level of Hyperventilation:

If a person's PMP is below 5 seconds, he is critically ill—whether he has symptoms or not. This child needs the immediate attention of a Breathing Normalization Specialist and a lot of one-on-one work.

The last line of the chart:

When a person passes away, his CP and PMP becomes zero.

Please note that an intake of steroids and other medical drugs can affect breathing measurements. Steroids always inflate CP and PMP. If your child is on steroids, keep in mind that his real measurements are significantly lower.

Also, the numbers in the chart above are accurate for locations at sea level. If a person is in a high altitude area, their numbers will be lower. For example, at a higher altitude, a PMP of 40 seconds could be equal to a PMP of 60 seconds at sea level, indicating that the person is in optimal health.

You probably noticed that there is also an **upper section in Buteyko's chart**. What happens when PMP goes above the norm? Is it even possible? Yes. Many of Dr. Buteyko's students had PMPs of

120 and even 180 seconds, and you, too, can train yourself or your child to get to that level. From Dr. Buteyko's perspective, this state of human well-being is extraordinary. High PMP certainly supports optimal health and longevity.

Please keep in mind the Breathing Normalization method is not a pill and will not change your child's health instantly. I've seen many people become impatient when they do not see instant results. It takes at least six months for the immune, nervous, and other bodily systems to rehabilitate themselves. The training facilitates this process, but there is no way to jump immediately from being an invalid to being superman. Recovery is gradual. Even though this method is the most effective and fastest healing technique I am familiar with, it still requires time. Nevertheless, you should be able to see some improvement in your child's asthma, which could be very significant, within a few weeks.

Healing Crisis
Parents need to be aware of the 'healing crisis' as their child recovers from hyperventilation. As the body moves toward balance, there usually comes a point at which symptoms increase or new symptoms appear. This is temporary, and it is a necessary step in the process of restoring health. This is very similar to a process which occurs in homeopathic and other holistic treatments.

Since the immune system has been weakened by the lack of oxygen, as it becomes stronger it attacks disease-causing microorganisms that were dormant in the body. This can result in fever, headache, upset stomach, intestinal upset or other ailments. These are symptoms of the strengthened immune system going after viruses and bacteria and expelling them from the body. They are temporary and are not cause for alarm.

On the path to recovery from hyperventilation, your child will most likely become ill once, twice, or in rare cases, a few times. Most likely the symptoms will appear the same as when your child has a cold or flu. It is important to let the child go through this process without suppressing the symptoms, if possible. It is a sign of the body's successful fight against disease and is required in order to restore health. It is fine to treat the illness with natural remedies if symptoms become bad enough. However, please try your best not to use chemically based medications unless it is necessary.

Also, during the healing crisis some asthma symptoms could temporarily become much stronger. Mucus and coughing could significantly increase for some children before they permanently weaken.

During a healing crisis, it is very important for the child to have plenty of rest and to stay warm and comfortable. If possible, keep your child out of school and away from intense physical exertion and over-excitement.

Usually the healing crisis does not last long—just a few days to a week—although in some cases it can extend to two weeks.

A healing crisis often occurs when the Control Pause reaches around 20 seconds. If your child's CP begins stabilizing at around 20 seconds, expect your child to temporarily feel ill, as he will likely go through a healing crisis at that time.

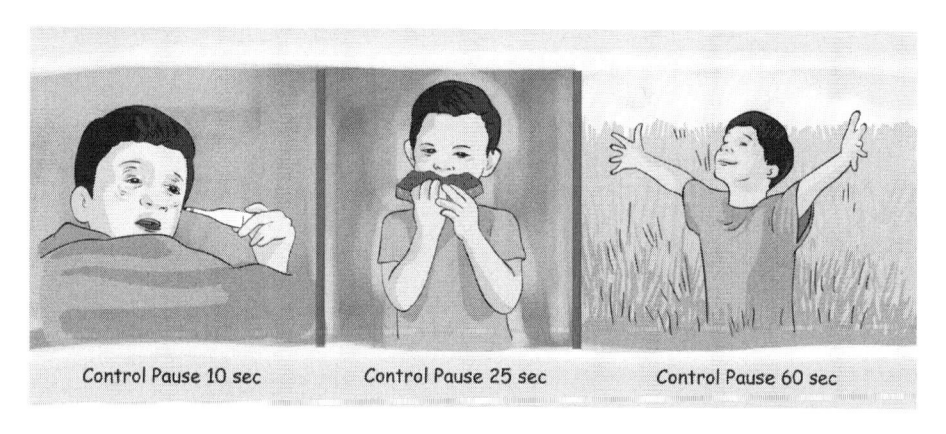

Control Pause 10 sec   Control Pause 25 sec   Control Pause 60 sec

How to recognize the healing crisis
A healing crisis can be confusing—it might look like a virus, suggesting that a child's health is getting poorer. It also could look as worsening of asthma and can be very concerning for parents. To differentiate the healing crisis from a disease state, you will need to

closely observe your child's breathing measurements. If his Morning Control Pause increases fast (for example, doubling within a couple of weeks), expect a healing crisis. When it starts, the Morning Control Pause will suddenly drop down and the child will not feel good. After the healing crisis is over, his Control Pause will rise again and will stabilize at a new, higher level.

A healing crisis can be scary, and yet it is a very positive event, one that normally brings an improved state of health. Explain this to your child so he can go through his healing crisis without worrying.

Part 2: Lifestyle Recommendations

If you are trying to stop your child's hyperventilation, an important factor to consider, besides obvious his or her breathing, is his or her lifestyle. Kids often have full schedules from dawn to dusk, leaving little time for play. Yes, many modern children play team sports, but this in itself is a competitive, stressful activity, and nothing like the free form of roaming around outdoors, which was the norm just one generation ago.

On top of this, children often consume too much food; their diet is not healthy, is too rich, and includes too many animal-based foods. They wear too many clothes, often made of synthetic materials; they live in a temperature-controlled environment, breathe polluted air, ride in cars and don't spend enough time outdoors. All these factors combined create an unnatural lifestyle that leads to unnatural breathing patterns.

But what are natural breathing patterns? According to Dr. Buteyko, when a child (or adult) is truly healthy, his breathing automatically pauses for a few seconds after every exhalation, instead of immediately continuing on to the next inhalation. Dr. Buteyko stated that this is the way wild animals breathe. Children in less developed countries whose lifestyle remains more natural often breathe like this. At Breathing Center, we teach parents to alter a child's lifestyle to a more natural healthier direction. As a result, a child develops a natural, automatic halt after exhalation.

Stress Reduction
Traditionally, children have had plenty of time to explore, to lie in the grass and look up at the clouds, to curl up in a chair and stare out the window, thinking of nothing or daydreaming, simply allowing their imagination to take them wherever it will.

These activities are relaxing. They serve as an antidote to stress. They are like pressing the reset button so that the system can start afresh.

Part 2: Lifestyle Recommendations by Sasha Yakovleva

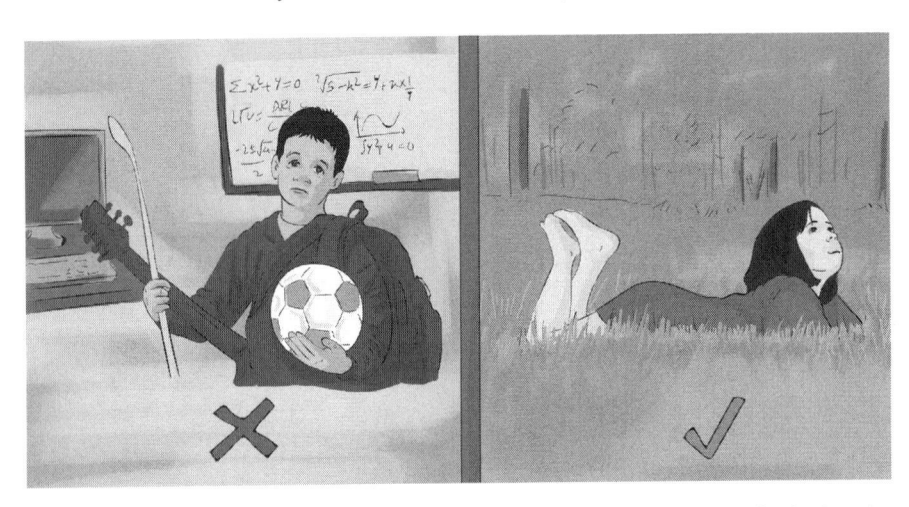

Many children today have practically every minute of their day scheduled: school, sports, classes after school, homework, etc. And when they do have time to themselves, they often spend it in front of a video screen shooting aliens or hunched over a handheld device texting. Such activities are not relaxing, but rather create more tension and stress.

When a child has time to truly relax, the breathing can settle down, and the body begins to move toward retaining sufficient carbon dioxide. This aspect is explored further in the *Breathing Exercises* part of this section of the book.

Breathing During Sleep
Since children are asleep for about one-third of each day, it is critical to address breathing issues during sleep. Nighttime breathing is usually even more excessive than daytime breathing. In addition, since we cannot consciously control over-breathing during sleep, sleeping encourages over-breathing.

Many children with asthma and other breathing problems sleep with their mouth open. Their respiration is loud and often accompanied by wheezing. They snore and often stop breathing for a while, eventually developing sleep apnea. They often wake up with a stuffy nose or throat and often start coughing right away. All these conditions are caused by over-breathing and can be stopped by light nasal breathing.

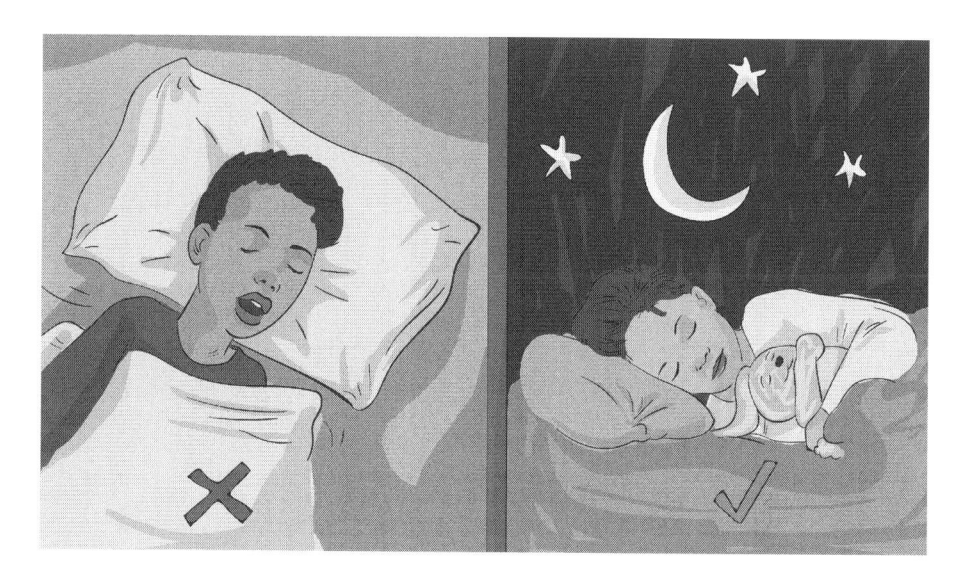

As with daytime practice, the goals of nighttime Breathing Normalization training are:

1. Establishing continuous nasal breathing
2. Reducing air consumption and air exchange.

Tape:
Establishing continuous nasal breathing at night is often achieved by using a gentle paper tape, which is available in most pharmacies. A small piece of this medical tape is placed on a child's lips, vertically, sealing the mouth. The tape acts as a reminder to keep the mouth closed, and encourages breathing through the nose. Although children often remove the tape in their sleep without realizing it, it provides at least a few hours of support for healthy breathing. Sleeping with the tape on through the whole night normally indicates that a child is capable of breathing exclusively through his nose through the night.

The idea of covering their mouth during sleep can be scary for some children. A good approach to this is to get the child used to wearing tape during the day and, as with so many elements of Breathing Normalization, to make it a family activity. The so-called *Tape Games*, described in the *Breathing Exercises* part of section of this book, are helpful aids. Once the child gets used to playing with tape during the day and feels comfortable having it on his lips, you can then experiment with using tape at bedtime.

I recommend that parents also use tape during sleep. This will not only benefit your own breathing, but will also help the child to see it as part of the family's daily health routine, like brushing teeth.

Anyone who uses tape during sleep long enough to become accustomed to it can attest to its benefits. Snoring and dry mouth become things of the past and sleep becomes more restful and rejuvenating. Children with asthma often stop wheezing and coughing at night because the tape prevents mouth breathing and greatly reduces hyperventilation. Children generally wake up in a better mood and with more energy.

Scarf:
Another tool—generally introduced after the child is comfortable with tape—is a lightweight scarf, preferably made of a natural fabric. Its purpose is to reduce air consumption during sleep. This is a useful tool for many children who over-breathe, but especially for those who have sleep apnea on top of asthma.

Wrap the scarf twice around the child's torso, just at the bottom edge of the rib cage, tight enough to keep the breathing in check, but without causing discomfort. Tie it with a knot in the back, so that if you see it come loose during the night, it's easy to re-tie without waking the child. Also, the knot in the back will prevent them from sleeping on their back, which can promote hyperventilation.

The scarf needs to be introduced gradually, first during waking hours, with the participation of the parents and the rest of the family whenever possible.

An asthmatic child could have a very negative reaction to the scarf because it might remind him of suffocation. If this is a case, never force a child to use the scarf. Breathing can be improved without this tool.

Other factors:
Many asthmatic children like to sleep face down—lying on their stomach and often hiding their face in a pillow. This position sometimes frightens parents because of a presumed risk of suffocation. In reality, sleeping on his stomach is the best position for a child's breathing. Breathing is naturally minimized by the child's own weight pressing on the diaphragm, and this helps keep hyperventilation in check. Many children intuitively like this position.

If a child is not comfortable sleeping on his stomach, the next best position for breathing is lying on the side with knees comfortably flexed.

The position to avoid is lying on the back, since this position promotes excessive breathing. In this position, the mouth often falls open, making nasal breathing impossible.

Also, a firm mattress and a firm, tall pillow are conducive to healthy breathing.

Eating a large, heavy meal before going to bed is not recommended. Excessive food, especially eaten late, provokes hyperventilation.

Physical Activity
Children often don't do enough physical activities. They spend many hours sitting in school, in front of the TV or at the computer. To compensate for this sedentary lifestyle, their parents organize various physical activities for them such as aerobics, tennis, soccer, etc. Often, these activities are short, but intense. This is very different from the lifestyle children had in the old days when they were physically active throughout the whole day, helping their parents with various chores and playing outside. The imbalance of physical activities is particularly dangerous for kids who have various breathing difficulties and specifically suffer from suffocation attacks.

It's a common belief that physical activities support health no matter what. But this isn't always true. If a child has a broken ankle, would you say that running is good for him? Of course not! It's the same with breathing—if a child's breathing is weak, strenuous physical activities only worsen his health. The difference between a broken ankle and "broken breathing" is that in the first case the problem is obvious, while in the second it is hidden, since "broken breathing" is not accompanied by bruises and pain. The "wound" remains unseen, and so is usually ignored by parents, who continue to insist that the child play sports without any consideration for how he feels.

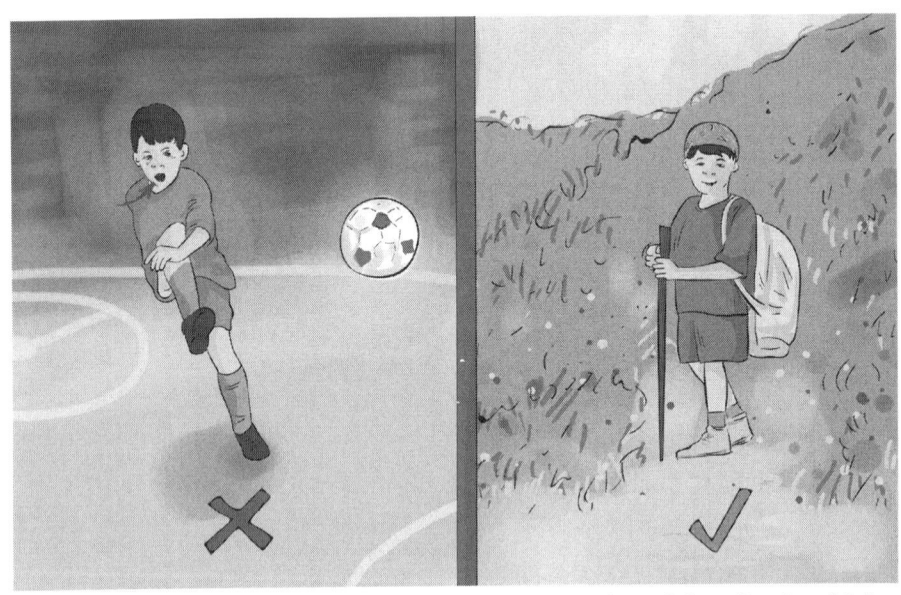

The first and <u>most important rule of physical activity</u>: It should be accompanied by nasal breathing only. Any physical exercise accompanied by mouth breathing can be damaging to the health of an asthmatic child.

At the beginning of the Breathing Normalization training, I ask parents to observe all their child's physical activities (especially team sports) and to discontinue them if those activities are accompanied by mouth breathing. This halt is only temporary; when their child's breathing becomes stronger, he can once again participate in the same physical activities. By then, those activities become beneficial. Over time, these physical activities (even team sports) can replace breathing exercises and become the main tool for continued breathing and health improvement. However, while the child's breathing is still weak, he needs to do breathing exercises to strengthen it to the point where he can handle workouts while breathing solely through the nose.

Once the child is capable of adequate nasal breathing, he can start participating in physical activities again. At that point, physical activities become important because, according to science, a body in motion actively generates CO2.

Among all possible physical activities, walking and running are most beneficial for breathing. Until very recently in human history, walking used to be an essential part of everyday life. Children walked to school, adults walked to work, and many people walked or stayed on their feet much of their workday. Now that we have cars and drive practically everywhere—at least in the United States—hardly anyone walks much. This is another contributor to hyperventilation, as walking is a relaxing, mild exercise, which tends to bring breathing back into balance. Any time you can take a walk with your child, take the opportunity. Walk at a pace that allows your child to breathe comfortably through the nose. If the child begins to breathe heavily, stop right away.

Diet

What to drink:
Breathing Normalization suggests drinking plenty of water of the purest quality you can find. It's the only liquid nature created for human consumption, so it is best to drink water only. Fresh, seasonal, organic juice is fine, too. Don't let your child drink sodas, caffeinated and vitamin drinks, or low quality bottled juices, since these drinks contain sugar and artificial additives.

What to Eat:
The best diet for asthmatic children is to eat organic, preferably local and seasonal foods, including plenty of vegetables, fruits, berries, grains, seeds and some nuts.

Part 2: Lifestyle Recommendations by Sasha Yakovleva

Dr. Buteyko recommends avoiding animal protein whenever you can. The typical diet with large amounts of animal protein is a serious contributor to hyperventilation. These products cause a reduction in Control Pause and often trigger symptoms. This is especially true for dairy products (particularly cheese), which generate excessive mucus. A piece of cheese alone could trigger an asthma attack. Various meats and poultry cause similar problems, as does fish, although to a lesser extent.

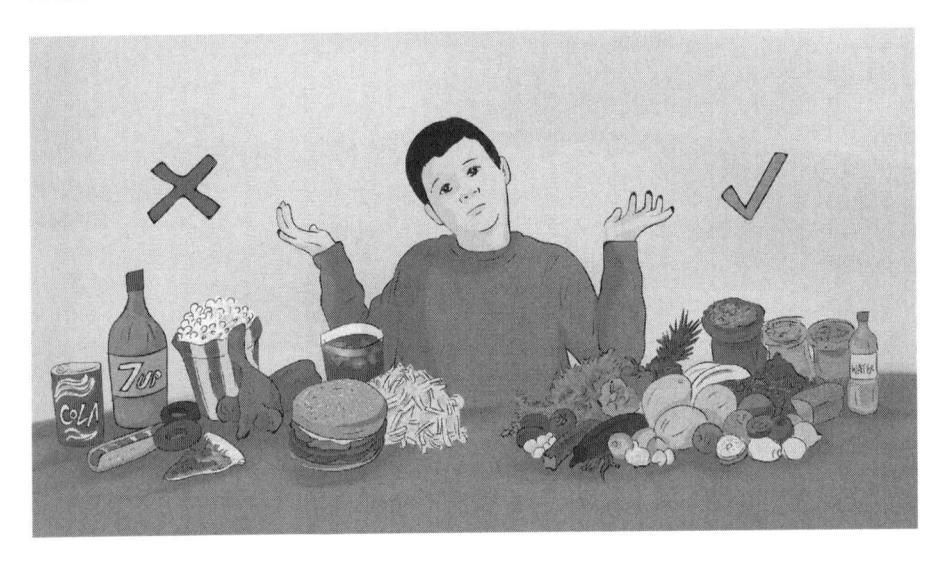

It is strongly suggested that during the process of Breathing Normalization the intake of all meats and dairy be greatly reduced or stopped completely. At the very least, make sure that your child does not eat animal-based products every day. Once the child significantly increases his Control Pause, the amount of animal products the child consumes can be reevaluated, but it is a key piece of the healing process while taming hyperventilation.

Junk foods should be cut out completely. Many children crave sweets. At the beginning of the breathing training it is often impossible to eliminate such cravings, but they do decrease when breathing—and metabolism—improves. Until then, try to replace candies containing artificial ingredients with fruits, maple syrup, honey and other naturally sweet products.

I don't recommend allowing children to chew gum. It doesn't benefit them, but it does distract them from maintaining awareness of their breathing.

Hunger:
One common misconception among parents is that a child must never feel hungry. Often, parents endlessly offer children snacks, sometimes encouraging them to take seconds at meals and eat more than they want to. Moderate hunger is not harmful; it positively contributes to breathing and health improvement. Conversely, overeating triggers hyperventilation. Never force a child to eat when he does not feel hungry.

Salt:
Some parents assume that salt should be avoided. For many years, salt had been demonized as a major cause of heart disease and heart attacks. However, recent studies have shown that this is not the case. From Dr. Buteyko's perspective, salt is an essential nutrient and should be part of the daily diet. People who hyperventilate often have mineral deficiencies. These can be restored naturally through salt intake. It is scientifically proven that good salt supports healthy metabolism, improves hydration, helps balance blood sugar and hormones, and is detoxifying.

I recommend using whole, unrefined sea salt—preferably *Himalayan salt* because it is pure and rich in minerals. Commercial table salt, bleached and stripped of minerals, does not, of course, benefit the body. Sea salts are much better, but unfortunately, they are polluted, since the oceans are filled with toxins. Himalayan salt, mined from ancient sea beds, is untainted by modern environmental toxins and provides a rich source of more than 80 trace minerals. Try to cook meals without salt and let members of your family, especially a child with asthma, add raw salt to their meals according to taste. In the beginning of their breathing training, some children have strong cravings for salt. If your child is one of them, don't worry about it. Let him eat as much salt as he wants. As his breathing improves, his salt consumption will naturally decrease.

Also, some children enjoy holding a salt crystal on their tongue until it dissolves. This can sometimes help reduce respiratory discomfort, especially when it is mucus-related. A glass of warm water with a little bit of Himalayan Salt dissolved in it can also be good for easing respiratory symptoms.

Nature
Spending time in nature is relaxing and healing, and is therefore a powerful antidote to hyperventilation. Fresh air is important for healthy breathing. Make sure that your child spends plenty of time outside.

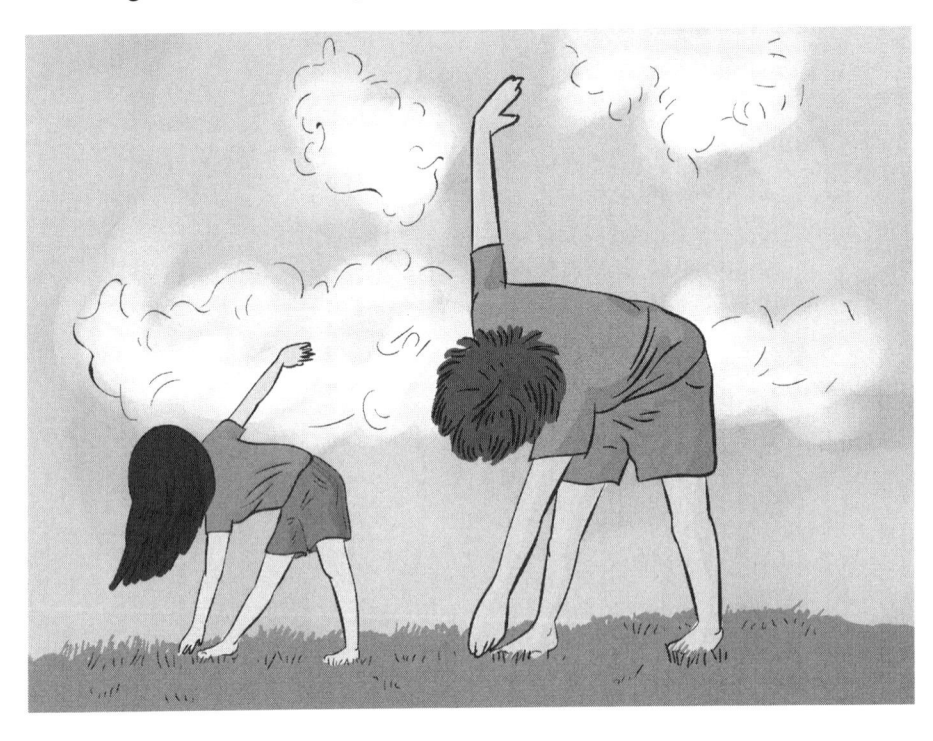

I also recommend keeping windows open in warm weather. When the weather turns cold, make a habit of opening windows frequently for a short time to let in fresh air. Especially when a child is sick, many parents tend to close all windows and keep the space hot. This is a bad idea—overheating always triggers hyperventilation. Numerous studies have shown that breathing cool, fresh air is most beneficial during active times as well as for rejuvenating sleep.

Excessive clothing also supports hyperventilation since it causes over-heating. Children don't like wearing hats, shoes and warm clothes, and parents often need to force the child to get dressed. If circumstances permit, allow your child to wear as few clothes as he wants, especially outside. Being exposed to cool, or even cold air and water, helps build strong immune, nervous and respiratory systems.

On the other hand, if a child's CP is below 10 to 15 seconds, he needs to be comfortable and warm. Cold temperatures, especially outdoors, can make his condition worse. For children with this condition, wrap a warm scarf around their mouth during cold winter weather to prevent them from breathing in cold air. Do breathing exercises with the child to strengthen his breathing and immune system. When his CP stabilizes above 15 seconds, you can gradually and carefully start exposing him to cold air and water.

The same is true for sunlight, which activates the metabolism and leads to more production of CO_2. Your child needs a lot of it, yet if his level of over-breathing is high, he may have very sensitive skin. He needs to be exposed to sunlight gradually. Be mindful, though, and if your child starts developing signs of sunburn or over-heating, take him inside immediately. Build his strength carefully and gradually, and by the end of summer your child will have a beautiful tan, which is a sign of good breathing and health.

Talking
People don't often realize that when they speak they inhale through their mouth. During Breathing Normalization training, we help people establish complete gentle nasal breathing while they talk. This may sound like a simple task, but it is actually the most challenging part of breathing training. It requires determination and a high level of awareness. Not all children are able to do it. Although nasal breathing while talking is not mandatory for children, it is highly recommended. If you help your child learn to breathe through his nose while talking, he will most likely retain this pattern for the rest of his life. This will protect him from the many health problems associated with mouth breathing, including viruses.

Part 2: Lifestyle Recommendations by Sasha Yakovleva

How should you or your child breathe while speaking? Gently inhale through your nose, talk on the exhalation, then pause, inhale through your nose again and continue. While this is simple, it's not easy and often requires months of training. If you'd like to learn how to do breathing exercises specifically for talking, I suggest watching *The Breathing Normalization Method* video training, available on our website on DVD or as a download.

Part 3: Breathing Exercises for Children

These exercises are recommended for children three years and older. With younger children, breathing should be improved primarily by following a lifestyle conducive to healthy breathing. Usually, a Breathing Normalization Specialist creates an individual program of breathing exercises tailored to the child's specific situation. For a parent who is not familiar with the breathing improvement work, doing the exercises correctly can be challenging. If you find yourself in this position, I recommend calling the Breathing Center, or emailing us to schedule at least one session with a Breathing Normalization specialist. Most sessions take place over Skype, an online video-calling program. During the session, a specialist will take breathing measurements, select appropriate exercises and personalize them for the child's individual situation. Working with a specialist helps parents create a program that will ensure the child's breathing and health will steadily improve.

Dr. Buteyko emphasized that breathing is very powerful; when done correctly, it strengthens health; when done incorrectly, it quickly impairs health. To avoid mistakes, I recommend parents practice a gentle approach while doing breathing exercises with their child. Keep in mind that if breathing exercises are done improperly, they can impair a child's health. Please exercise mindfulness and caution.

During breathing exercises, a child should keep his lips completely closed and breathe exclusively through his nose. If a child is not able to breathe through his nose, stop the exercise or decrease its intensity. Do the same if you notice increasing signs of hyperventilation, such as noisy breathing, wheezing, or excessive movements of the shoulders, chest or stomach.

- Breathing exercises should not be done on a full stomach. It is always better to do them before a meal.
- Breathing exercises may be done formally in a structured session, or informally throughout the day.

I recommend that a child do three sessions a day—in the morning (before school), in the afternoon (after school) and before dinner or bedtime. Each session takes 30 minutes and often starts with 5 minutes of relaxation, followed by breathing exercises either in a seated position or in motion.

On top of the formal sessions, I recommend doing breathing exercises informally, whenever possible—in the car, on a walk, at recess, in front of the TV, etc. It is important to know how to check the effectiveness of the breathing exercises. There are two indicators: how the child feels and the breathing measurements.

Always carefully observe the child's breathing after a formal session of breathing exercises. Make sure that it has become less pronounced. Ask your child how he is feeling. Also, ask the child to imagine his breathing patterns as ocean waves. You can ask, "Are the waves stormy, wild or peaceful?" If the exercises are done properly, the waves will be peaceful, and the child will always breathe easily and feels better after.

Your observations combined with how your child says he feels provide you with valuable data. However, objective data is needed as well. This can be obtained by taking breathing measurements. To evaluate the results of a formal exercise session, measure your child's Control Pause before and after each session. The pre-session Control Pause is taken in a seated position right before the session. With a session of exercises in motion, the post-session Control Pause should be taken 15 to 30 minutes after the session, once the child's breathing has calmed. If the child was sitting or standing still during the session, the post-session Control Pause should be taken 3 to 5 minutes after the session. In both cases, the child should not eat anything or do anything physically strenuous; otherwise, the post-session Control Pause measurement will be incorrect. The Control Pause after the session should always be higher than the Control Pause before the session. If it is lower, then the exercises were done incorrectly, or perhaps the session was too long, too intense, or not challenging enough. Something will need to be changed in order for the exercises to become effective. The necessary change will vary for each individual and each situation. This is where input from an experienced Breathing Normalization specialist is especially valuable.

Another objective measurement of a child's progress, and perhaps an even more important one, is his Morning Control Pause. A steady increase in the Morning Control Pause indicates that his breathing exercises, both formal and informal, are effective. Since there is no immediate way to check the result of an informal exercise, we can evaluate it only approximately by relying on the Morning Control Pause.

Sometimes, parents aren't sure how to select the right breathing exercises. Normally, a breathing specialist determines the specific exercises that are appropriate for a particular child. I recommend trying all the exercises, or most of them, to determine which ones work best for your child. Pick ones he likes best and those that yield the biggest increase in his Control Pause. Once you have determined the best mix of exercises, let your child practice them for a while. When a child's Control Pause has increased by 5 to 10 seconds, test the exercises again and select new ones if necessary.

A child's breathing improvement greatly depends on the determination, commitment and involvement of his parents or guardians. And even though a parent has to lead the breathing normalization process, to be successful he must also relate to the child as an equal. It never works when a parent tells his child, "You hyperventilate; you are ill; you must do your breathing exercises to get healthy, and I will teach them to you!" The child should not feel like he is ill and weak, while everyone around is just fine. The way to guarantee a child's progress is to set things up as an equal partnership between you and your child from the start. Begin by explaining to your child that correct breathing is essential for health, so the whole family is going to work on improving their breathing together. To work on this, the parents as well as the child (and also possibly his brothers and sisters) are going to do breathing exercises (play breathing games) to help each other.

For parents who have never had breathing difficulties and have never had to struggle to breathe only through the nose, it can be an eye-opening experience to realize how difficult it is to change a mouth breathing habit. Also, don't be surprised if your child's Control Pause soon surpasses your own. It is often easier for children to establish natural breathing patterns than it is for their parents.

One of the pitfalls of parents working with children is that there is sometimes a tendency for them to criticize their child when he breathes incorrectly. Avoid criticism at all costs, because even if the child complies with the correction, being criticized will stress the child, which will increase his hyperventilation and defeat the whole purpose of working on improving the breathing. The most effective way to encourage healthy breathing is through positive reinforcement.

Instead, create circumstances in which the child experiences a sense of success. At the beginning of a first session with a child, I often say to him or her, "I need your help! My memory is not that great, and I often forget to breathe through my nose. Any time you notice me breathing through my mouth, please say, 'Sasha, stop breathing through your mouth! It's bad for your health! Remember, breathe through your nose only!'" Throughout the session, I periodically open my mouth and take in air in a deliberately noisy way. The child is always delighted to catch me doing this. I recommend that parents play the same game at home.

Kids love correcting their parents! It's essential that the child experience success. Let your child catch you in a mistake and accept his correction. Without this, the child can feel resentful and put-upon, which can hold up his breathing improvement. So, when your child catches you in a mouth breath, enthusiastically thank him. A positive approach helps children feel good and keeps them eager to continue Breathing Normalization.

It creates a positive context for you to correct your child when you see him breathing through his mouth. What could otherwise be a sensitive moment instead becomes just a part of the breathing game and another success. A light, fun tone is helpful. If you say, "Uh oh, there you go again. Why can't you learn to keep your mouth shut?" you'll get nowhere. Instead say, "Wow! I just saw you breathing through your mouth. I'm glad I'm not the only one who sometimes does that! Good thing I noticed it; now you can switch to healthy nose breathing."

It's crucial for the parent to realize that when a child breathes through the mouth, it's not a failure. It's an opportunity to learn to breathe better. The child has been breathing through his mouth for a while, possibly even his entire life, so, it will take time to develop an entirely new habit.

Don't forget to reward a child for his hard work and achievements. Let's say that for a week, your six-year-old son has had the discipline to do three formal sessions of breathing exercises a day. Acknowledge his success by treating him to his favorite activity. I always recommend that parents give their child a little present when his Control Pause jumps up to the next 5-second range.

I. Breathing Exercises in a Still Position:

I recommend starting Breathing Normalization training by doing this segment of breathing exercises first. Exercises in a motionless position might be slightly boring for an active child, but you can make them more appealing by rewarding the child for his achievements. These still exercises are necessary because they help develop breathing awareness, which is the foundation from which one can modify their breathing. Without this base, doing breathing exercises in motion can be problematic.

1. Do I Breathe Through my Mouth?

A parent and a child catch each other when one breathes though the mouth. This exercise is described in the first section of this chapter and is repeated below.

During breathing exercises, a child should keep his lips completely closed and breathe exclusively through his nose. If a child is not able to breathe through his nose, stop the exercise or decrease its intensity. Do the same if you notice increasing signs of hyper-ventilation, such as noisy breathing, wheezing, or excessive movements of the shoulders, chest or stomach.

This is an informal exercise.

2. American Indian Mother

Anthropologists have observed that indigenous peoples who live close to the land and have not been influenced by industrialization know the importance of minimal, nasal breathing. From birth, children are trained to not breathe through the mouth. When a mother sees her child with his mouth open, she gently closes the child's mouth using two fingers. This is done both while children are asleep as well as when they are active.

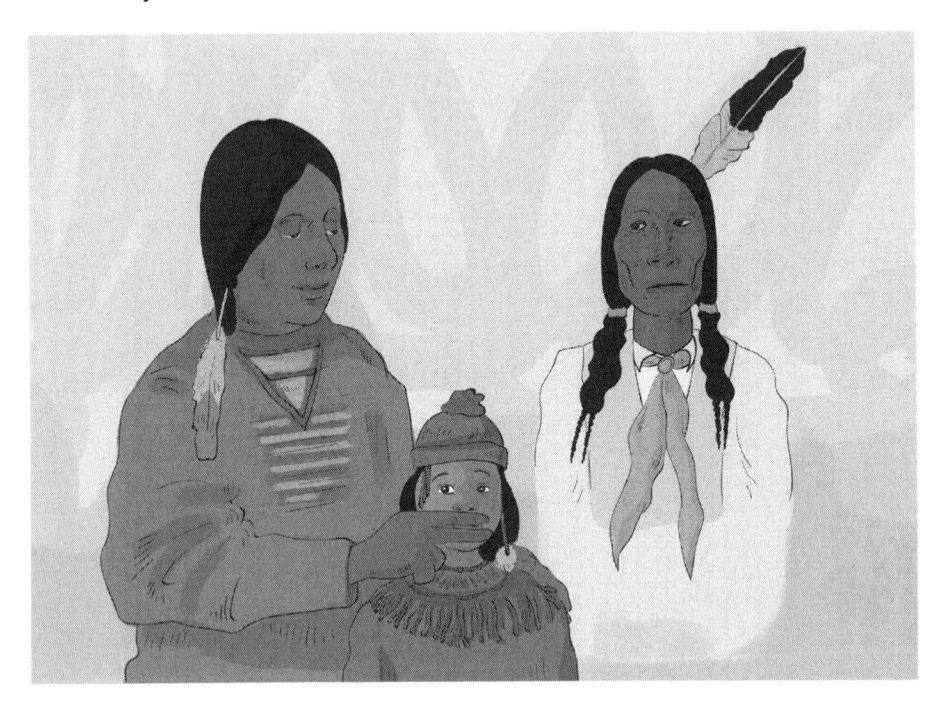

This is a method that has to be employed care-fully and with a lot of awareness on the part of the parent. A child might feel violated if, out of the blue, their parents start reaching over and closing his mouth at odd moments. This should be done lovingly, mostly as a gentle reminder that the mouth is supposed to remain closed except during eating and talking.

The best approach, again, is to make it into a game and communicate on an equal level. Explain to the child that this is part of the whole family learning to breathe correctly, and that the child should help the parent in the same way. It has to be done with a feeling of joy and fun, not impatience or condemnation. If a child feels stressed, his stress will promote hyperventilation and defeat the purpose of any breathing exercise. Always remember that relaxation is very important for healthy breathing.

This is an informal exercise.

3. Show Me Your Breathing

This exercise does not directly contribute to breathing improvement, but for many children, especially very young ones, it's an essential prerequisite to their breathing training.

Some small children don't realize that they breathe and are unable to distinguish between inhalation and exhalation, so this exercise is designed to make sure that they can.

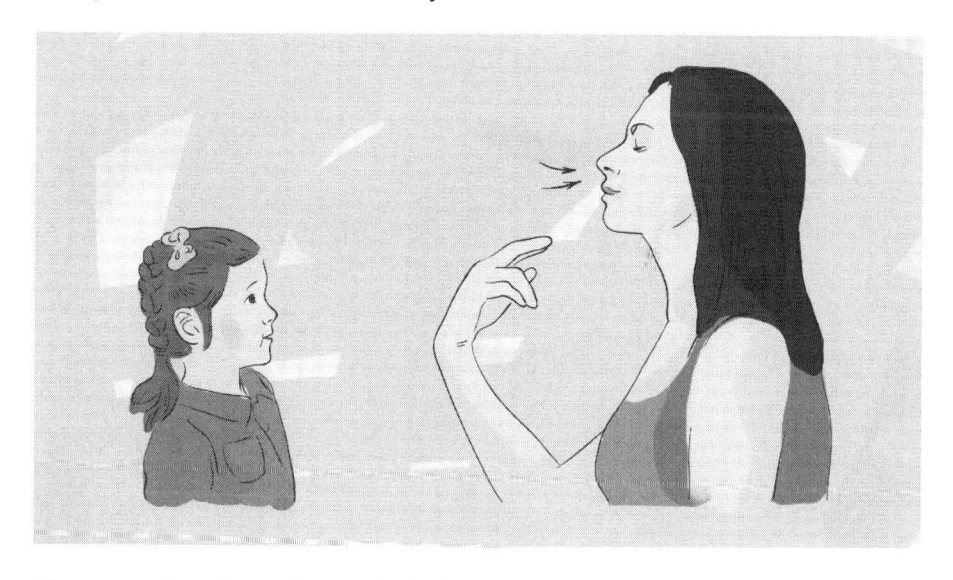

Use your hand to show inhalation and exhalation, moving it toward and away from your face, to match each inhale and exhale. Then, have the child do the same. If he is confused about it, continue to demonstrate and coach him until he is able to match the movement of his hand with the direction of the breath: inhale, move hand toward the mouth; exhale, move hand away.

This exercise is often done at the beginning of a session. It is also helpful just before a child starts to do breath holds.

This is an informal exercise. Duration: 1 to 3 minutes.

4. Are my Shoulders/Chest/Stomach Moving?

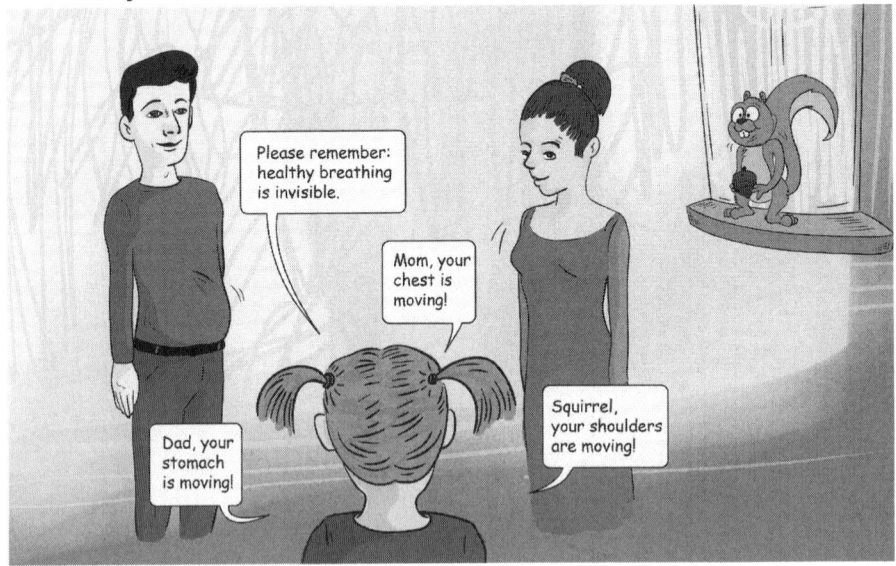

Again, a noticeable movement of any part of the body triggered by breathing—while a person is still—is an indicator of hyperventilation. Ask your child:

- Are your shoulders moving?
- Is your chest moving?
- Is your belly moving?

Once the error is pointed out, a child should practice light breathing with no excessive movement. Parent and child can take turns coaching each other. This is another good opportunity for the parent to deliberately make mistakes, so the child can point them out. It's good if the parent is corrected first, so the child will then feel happier and more comfortable when receiving a correction from the parent.

To do this exercise, the child needs to be still, preferably sitting on a hard chair with a straight back. Make sure the child sits up straight. The child can put one hand on his stomach and another on his chest to check if his shoulders, chest and stomach are moving. At the beginning of Breathing Normalization training, it is impossible for most children—as well as most adults—to stop excessive body movements; however, they can reduce them. Bear in mind that this is a gradual process, and success will come by degrees. The first step is to increase awareness of excessive body movements.

And to reduce such movements? Breathe slower and gentler!

Most of the time this exercise is done during a formal session, but it can also be done informally. Duration: 5 to 10 minutes.

5. Is my Breathing Noisy?

Audible breathing is an indication of over-breathing, or hyper-ventilation. This exercise is one of the elements of breathing that can be an ongoing game for the whole family. Players point out noisy breathing to each other. It's especially important for the parent to remember to thank the child for his correction.

Ask your child, "Can you hear your breathing?"

Once awareness is brought to noisy breathing, a child needs to make the effort to breathe slower and gentler and to relax, so that the breathing quiets down. Healthy breathing is not audible.

This is an informal exercise; however, it should be performed during a session if the child's breathing suddenly becomes noisy.

6. Book on the Belly

Have the child lie on his back with his head supported so it's easy for him to see his belly. Have him place a book on his belly and observe whether it's moving with each breath. The goal is to have the book move as little as possible. This teaches light, gentle, healthy breathing—the opposite of hyperventilation. Remember that healthy breathing is invisible.

Also, ask the child to stop the book from moving for 1 to 2 seconds after an exhalation. If the book stops moving even for one second, acknowledge this as an achievement. It is not easy to stop belly movements from a horizontal position. Try to do this exercise on your own before introducing it to your child.

This is a formal exercise but can be used informally. Duration: 3 to 5 minutes.

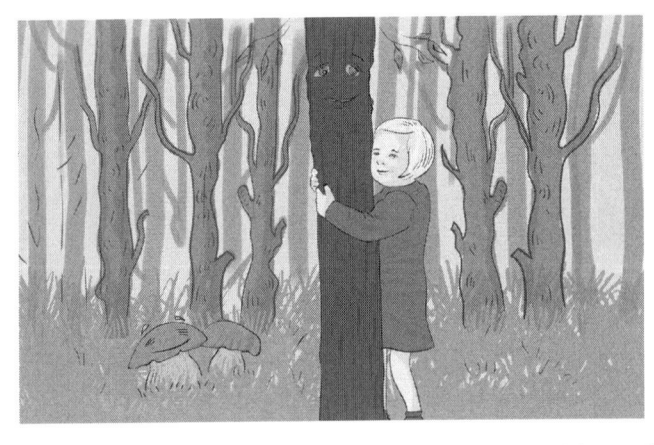

7. Hug a Tree

Instead of using a book, use a tree trunk to observe a child's stomach movements. While on a walk, ask the child to hug a tree and gently push his torso into the trunk. Make sure that the child's stomach, chest and shoulders don't move; that his breathing is light and quiet. Remember, a child with enlarged adenoids can only do this when he is relaxed.

Informal exercise. Duration: 3 to 5 minutes.

8. A little Mouse

This is one of the best-known Buteyko exercises. Originally, Dr. Buteyko created it for children, but adults, especially those suffering from asthma, have also found it useful.

Tell a child to imagine that Asthma is a giant cat hiding behind a curtain. The cat is watching the child, and if it can see or hear the child breathe, it will pounce and catch him or her. To win, the child must breathe quietly and invisibly (with the mouth closed, shoulders, chest and stomach still) so that the cat won't pounce.

This exercise can be done both formally and informally. It is often used to stop symptoms triggered by hyperventilation.

Duration: 5 to 10 minutes.

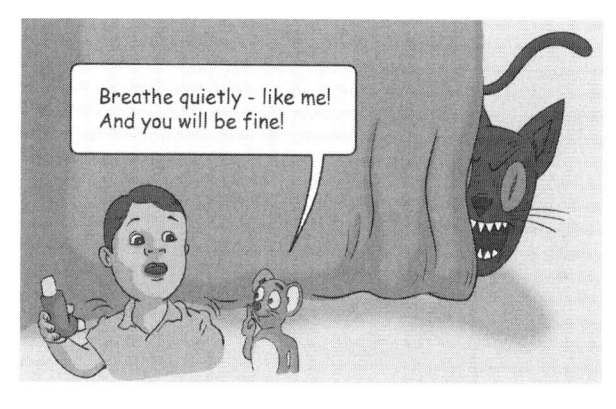

9. Be a Samurai

In ancient Japan, a feather was sometimes used to check if an aspiring samurai was breathing gently enough to thereby qualify to be a warrior. The feather was placed under a boy's nose; if he could breathe without moving the feather, he would be accepted. This test might sound strange to most, but it makes total sense to those familiar with Breathing Normalization. Only a person whose health is perfect (on a physical, emotional and psychological level) is capable of breathing without moving the feather.

This same test could be used as a breathing exercise for a child with asthma. The game is to hold a feather under the nose and breathe so gently that it moves as little as possible. The advantage of this exercise is that the effects of the breath can be clearly seen.

An alternative is to put a finger under the nose instead of a feather. In this version, the child can feel the flow of his breath instead of seeing it move the feather.

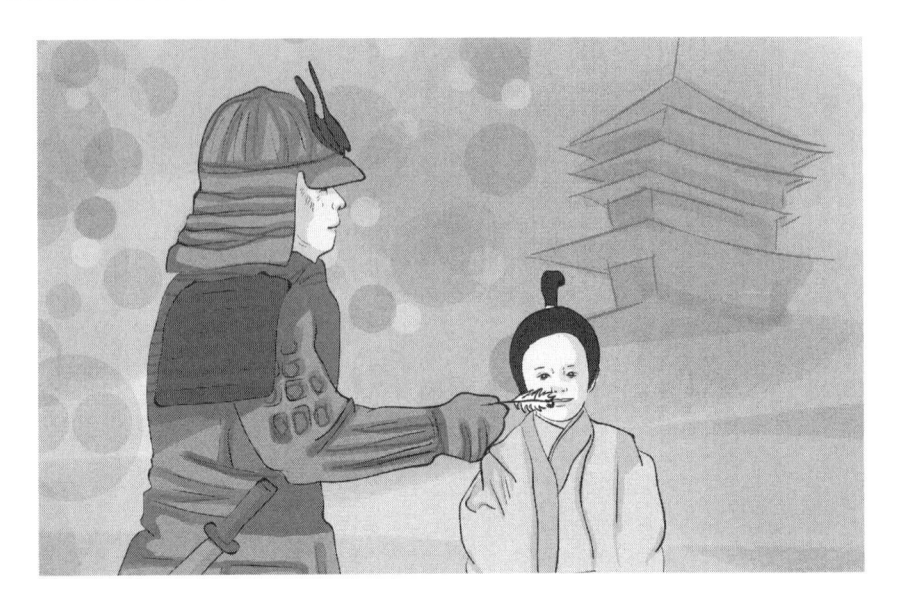

This exercise could be done both during a session and informally. Duration: 1 to 5 minutes.

10. Tape Exercises
Adults who practice the Breathing Normalization method often sleep with a small piece of medical tape attached across the upper and lower lips. This keeps the mouth closed and prevents snoring, mouth dryness, and most importantly, hyperventilation. At first, this can be challenging or scary. To get children comfortable using the tape at night, start by incorporating it into a game during the day. Aside from preparing a child for using the tape at night, daytime tape games have another purpose: to bring awareness to the lips, which is **important in establishing complete nasal breathing.**

For these exercises, use only gentle medical paper tape.

A) No Semi-Smile

Many children who hyperventilate almost never close their lips entirely. Often, they keep their lips slightly opened, forming them into what could be called a "semi-smile." You may have seen this look on a child's face and thought, "How cute." It might look cute, but it promotes mouth breathing. To teach a child to keep his lips closed, you will need to use tape.

Many children who hyperventilate almost never close their lips entirely. Often, they keep their lips slightly opened, forming them into what could be called a "semi-smile." You may have seen this look on a child's face and thought, "How cute." It might look cute, but it promotes mouth breathing. To teach a child to keep his lips closed, you will need to use tape.

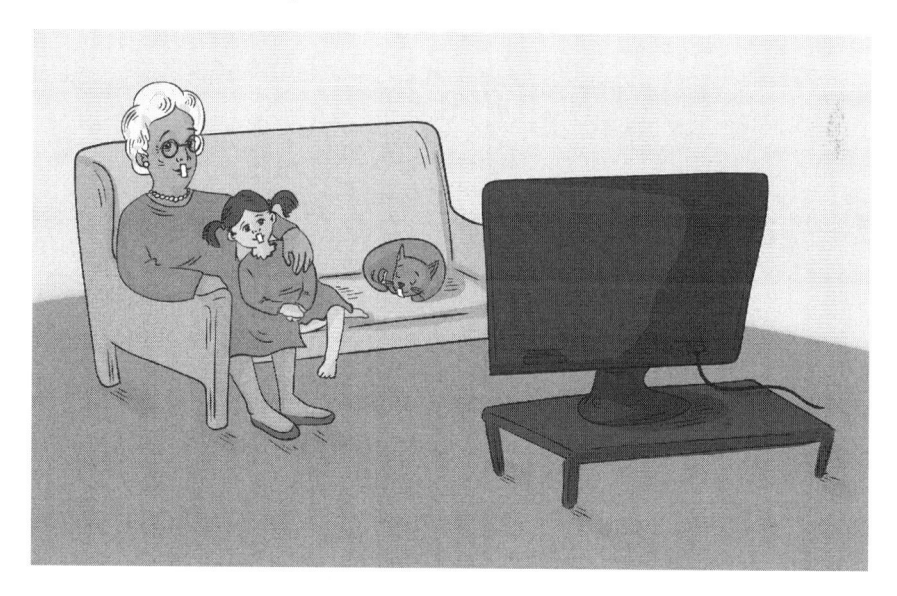

Another exercise is for the parent and child to wear tape around the house, removing it only when one of you needs to speak. Put a little piece of tape over your mouth, vertically, keeping your lips completely closed. Have the child do the same. Take the tape off any time you need to say something; put it back right after you stop talking. Your child should do the same any time he talks. Many children who hyperventilate are very talkative, and on top of that, they have no awareness of when their speech starts and ends. Because of that, it is difficult for them to put the tape back on when they finish a sentence. This game helps them develop the awareness to close their mouth after they finish speaking. This is an informal exercise.

B) Who Can Do it Longer?

The parent and the child sit together (perhaps while watching TV), each with a small piece of tape over the mouth. The game is to see who can keep the tape on the longest.

This game teaches a child to keep his lips completely closed for a long period of time. It also allows the child to be silent for an extended period, which is good for breathing. This is informal exercise.

---

11. Nose Songs

Nose Songs are a fun way to reduce breathing and counteract hyperventilation. The parent can demonstrate by making up a silly melody, while humming only through the nose. The child can add to it or make up his own song.

Ask the child to create a happy melody, and then make up a sad song—which can be just as silly and fun as the happy song. Try to awaken the child's creativity so the breathing exercises are joyful. Have fun together!

The benefit of this exercise is not only nasal breathing, but also a longer exhalation, which reduces air intake and increases the carbon dioxide level. Why? Because when we are exhaling, we cannot inhale at the same time. A long exhalation reduces the number of inhalations per minute and therefore increases the level of CO_2.

Remember to inhale through the nose only. The mouth should remain closed.

This exercise can be done formally or informally. Duration: 3 to 7 minutes.

12. Polly's Angel

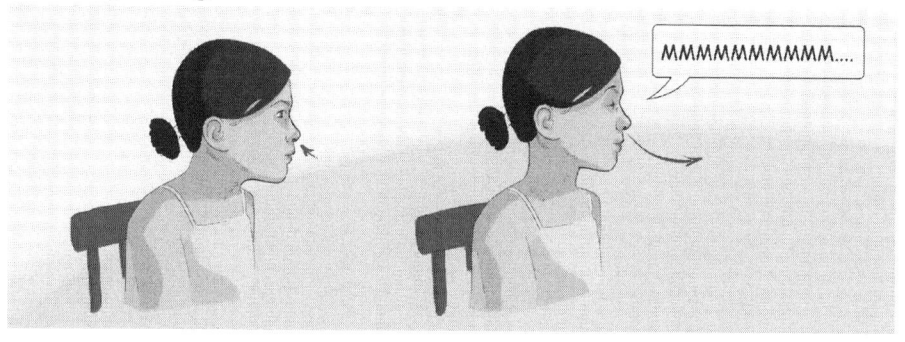

This exercise is named after Polly, a little girl who had severe asthma. She was taking various medications but none that would take away her breathing difficulties. She came up with her own solution by accident. Polly found that when she hummed a long monotone sound, she felt better. Because it was the only thing that made her feel better, she came to the conclusion that it was an angel making this sound to help her feel better.

Of course, knowing Dr. Buteyko's discovery, we can say that a sustained exhalation curbs hyperventilation and reduces symptoms that act as defense mechanisms against it. For a child with asthma, this effect is usually immediately obvious. Keeping the mouth closed and humming for a long period greatly reduces breathing, so it is helpful to children who over-breathe.

This exercise is usually done informally, but can be included in a formal session. Duration: 3 to 5 minutes.

13. A Sophisticated Device

Today's marketplace offers various breathing devices, the purpose of which is to force a person to breathe less by restricting the flow of air. These devices can bring momentary relief. However, they don't change a person's overall condition because they don't foster awareness of mouth, and they don't provide breathing modification aids. They often promote mouth breathing. Yet, many people are tempted by breathing devices because they seem like an easy solution. Well, you already have a simple solution. One sophisticated breathing reduction device is always with you: your fingers. By using a finger, you can easily achieve the same effect as that of some well-known breathing devices. There is a variety of ways to do this:

- Block one nostril by pressing on it with a finger or two. Make sure that your breathing does not become forceful or audible, and alternate the nostril you block. Congratulations! You just cut your air consumption in half!

- If the exercise above is too difficult, press on both nostrils lightly. Apply a bit of pressure, and then release your fingers to determine the minimum airflow that feels bearable to you. Adjust the pressure so it feels comfortable.

- Another alternative is to use the pad of your finger to partially block the opening of one or both nostrils. You are in control of your airflow—adjust it by moving your finger.

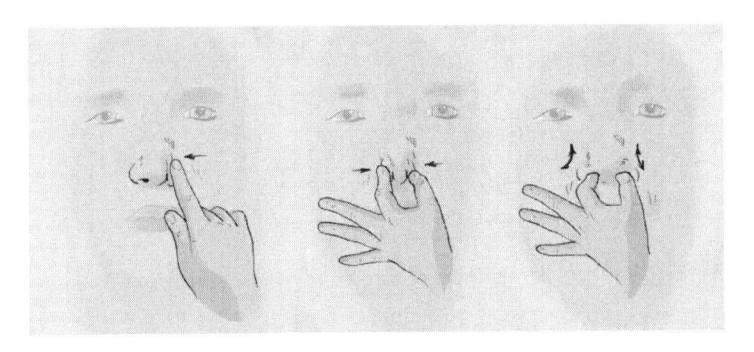

We recommend that parents do these exercises first and then teach their child how to do them. Please keep in mind that for a child with enlarged adenoids this particular exercise might be very difficult! Parents need to be patient and practice a gentle approach.

I recommend starting this as a formal exercise. Once the child is comfortable practicing it, it can be done informally. Duration: 3 to 5 minutes.

14. Fixed Breath Holds

This exercise is practiced in a seated position. Use a hard chair with a hard back. Divide your child's pre-session Control Pause by 3 to determine the number of seconds he can comfortably go without air. For example, if the pre-session Control Pause is 15 seconds, use 5 seconds for the breath holds. Ask your child to block his nose using his fingers for 5 seconds following an exhale. You will need to count the seconds out loud, so he knows how close he is to the end of a breath hold. This will help him to feel more in control. Once the breath hold is finished, make sure the child gently inhales through his nose. Repeat a breath hold of 5 seconds every minute. Use this minute in between breath holds as a break for the child to breathe normally, calmly, and only through the nose.

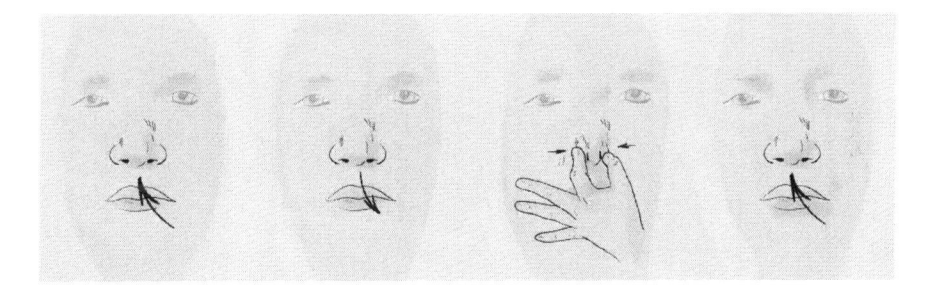

Breath holds must be done only AFTER exhalation, NOT after inhalation.

This is a formal exercise. Duration: 5 to 30 minutes. Do not exceed 30 minutes.

15. Flexible Breath Holds

This exercise is the same as a *Fixed Breath Hold*, except that the duration of the breath holds is not fixed. Based on a child's Control Pause, determine the number of seconds he can comfortably go without air. For example, if the pre-session Control Pause is 15 seconds, the duration of the first breath hold should be 5 seconds. Ask the child to block his nose with his fingers for 5 seconds after an exhalation and then slowly start to increase the duration of the breath holds.

For example, the first breath hold is 5 seconds. Repeat it three times, with a minute between each breath holds. Then, ask your child to do a 6-second breath hold. Carefully observe the child's breathing during and after each breath hold. If there are no signs of hyperventilation, continue with the 6-second breath hold for up to three times. If there are still no signs of hyperventilation, try 7 seconds; do it three times, then try 8 seconds. If at any moment your child hyperventilates, let him rest until he stops over-breathing, then switch back to shorter breath holds. For example, if the child's breathing becomes loud at the 8-second breath hold, let him rest quietly for 5 minutes, then continue with three 5-second breath holds before starting to build up the time again. Alternately, just switch to *Fixed Breath Holds* and continue doing 5-second breath holds for the remainder of the session. Breath holds should be done only AFTER exhalation, NOT after inhalation.

This is a formal exercise. I recommend doing this exercise for 5 to 30 minutes; do not exceed 30 minutes.

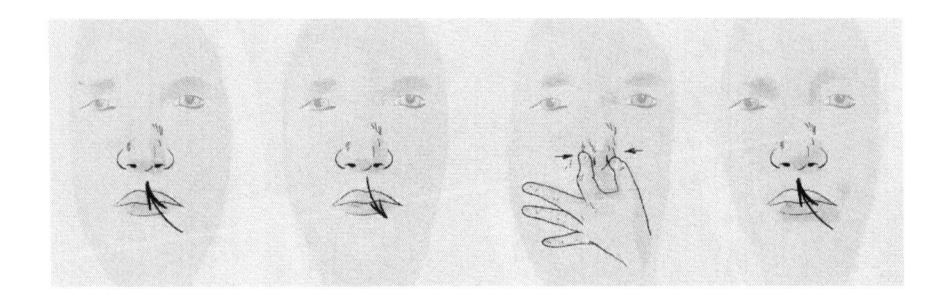

II. Breathing Exercises in Motion

Breathing exercises in motion are more effective than still exercises. However, they can also be dangerous if done incorrectly. Be sure to follow the instructions precisely. The exercises below are listed from the easiest to the most challenging. I recommend starting with the easiest ones.

16. Airplane

This exercise is a variation on *Polly's Angel*. Ask the child to extend his arms and pretend to fly around the room like an airplane, while imitating the various hums of a plane engine.

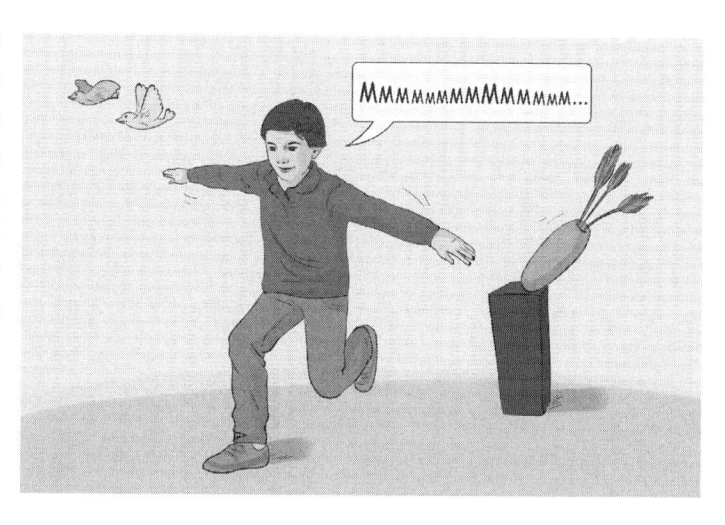

The mouth should remain closed, with nasal inhalation only. The movements should be slow and gentle.

This exercise is mostly used informally; if used formally, I recommend adding it to the beginning or end of a formal session.

Duration: 3 to 10 minutes.

17. Dancing with a Nose Song

Movement in combination with nasal breathing helps alleviate hyperventilation. When movement and nasal breathing are combined with humming, they become an even more effective tool against hyperventilation. Dance with your child while simultaneously humming nose songs. Have fun! Make sure your child does not move fast; he should inhale only through the nose.

This exercise is mostly used informally; if used formally, I recommend adding it to the beginning or end of a formal session.

Duration: 3 to 10 minutes.

18. Walking, Hiking, Running

Long walks are one of the best ways to improve breathing and end hyperventilation. Traditionally, long walks were a part of a child's life, but our car-centric culture has changed this. Modern kids are often driven to school, as well as to after-school activities; they don't spend hours playing outside as their parents or grandparents did. The resulting sedentary lifestyle is one of the main causes of hyperventilation. Often, kids are incapable of walking even for thirty minutes. If your child is one of them, you need to start building endurance.

~ Walking

Walk with your child for as long as his breathing allows. The child must breathe through his nose the whole time. This means that he needs to be quiet while walking, or only speak when necessary. If your child's breathing becomes loud or he starts to feel that he needs to open his mouth, slow your walking pace or stop completely to let your child rest. If the child begins gasping, or cannot keep his mouth closed, stop immediately and rest until his breathing returns to normal. If your child's hyperventilation is severe, begin with short walks.

~ Hiking

Slow, long walks at a stable pace combined with all health benefits nature offers is incredibly healing for breathing. Take your child for long hikes as often as possible. Make sure that your child breathes exclusively through his nose. Build your child's hike endurance slowly and gradually. Be patient!

~ Running

Slow jogging at a consistent pace is also a very effective healing technique. Most children who have asthma aren't able to run while quietly breathing through their noses at the start of their Breathing Normalization training. Once it becomes easy for a child to walk and do breath holds (see instructions for Steps With Breath Holds (number 21, following), he can start running.

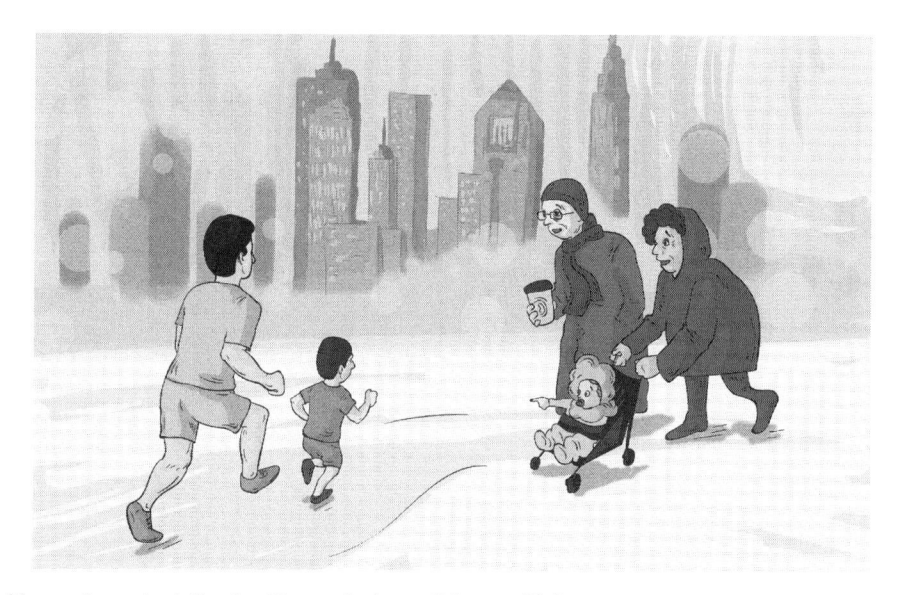

Keep in mind that although breathing will become more pronounced and noticeable during running, it needs to remain quiet. If it becomes heavy and noisy, stop the exercise or ask your child to walk until his breathing normalizes.

I recommend that parents purchase a treadmill for in-home exercise. This allows a child to practice breathing in motion, regardless of weather conditions, anytime he has an extra 10 or 20 minutes. If a child spends several hours doing his homework, it is important for his health to take walking or running breaks. Make sure that his mouth remains closed. Sometimes, a little piece of tape is helpful in keeping the lips closed.

If a treadmill is not an option, I recommend using a jump rope. The child's mouth should remain closed during jumping. Some parents use a trampoline for the same purposes; however, it is much more difficult to control breathing on a trampoline. Some children end up hyperventilating after jumping on a trampoline—it can be too exciting, making light breathing difficult. These are very effective informal activities.

Part 3: Breathing Exercises for Children by Sasha Yakovleva

19. Don't Miss the Fridge

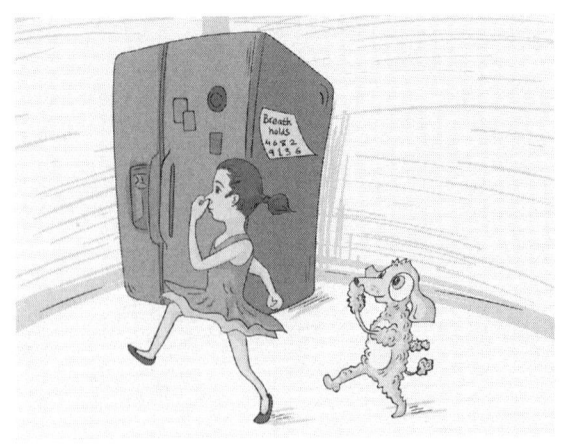

Designate a large object somewhere in the house, say a fridge or a table, and ask your child to do a breath hold every time he passes by the object. The breath hold can be two or three seconds, nothing extreme. This keeps bringing attention back to the breath and balances it by limiting breathing for a few moments.

You will need to participate in this exercise, too, so that it feels like a fun game for your child. You can even keep score! Delight your child by letting him catch you occasionally forgetting to do a breath hold when you walk by the fridge.

This exercise should be done periodically; it is used only informally.

20. A Corner-to-Corner Walk with Breath Holds
This is a more advanced exercise, or game, and should be given only after the child has reached a consistent Control Pause of 15 seconds.

Ask, "Can you go from one corner of the room to the opposite one without breathing at all?"

If he says yes, ask him to go ahead and do it. Observe carefully to be sure that once breathing resumes, there is no gasp on the inhalation. If there is, go to a smaller room or try an easier exercise!

Breath holds should be done ONLY after exhalation, NOT after inhalation.

This exercise may be used formally or informally.

Duration: I recommend doing this exercise for 5 to 10 minutes. Make sure the child has about a 2-minute break between breath holds to breathe normally and relax.

21. Steps with Breath Holds

Sometimes, I meet children who learned this particular Buteyko exercise from someone who is not authorized to teach Buteyko Breathing Normalization. The results are often negative and make the child feel worse. That's because instructions from unauthorized sources often suggest combining steps with a maximum length of breath holds. This actually strengthens hyperventilation and discourages healthy breathing!

Ask your child to walk around. He should start by taking soft steps; if his breathing allows, later in the exercise he can make his steps more pronounced by lifting his legs higher and stepping down forcefully.

Next, ask your child to do a breath hold while walking. The breath hold should be easy—around 2 seconds. When the breath hold is finished, the child should continue walking in the manner described above for about 2 minutes. Then, repeat the same length breath hold. If the child does not display signs of hyperventilation, start increasing the length of the breath holds by 1 second at a time, and continue doing breath holds every 2 minutes. Never ask your child to do a maximum breath hold. Breathing Normalization requires a gentle approach. Straining only produces negative results.

Breath holds should be done ONLY after exhalation, NOT after inhalation.

This is an excellent exercise to use during a formal session.

Duration: 5 to 30 minutes. Do not exceed 30 minutes.

22. Walk with Breath Holds

Walking to school or to the bus stop is a perfect opportunity for breathing exercises. While walking, the child holds his breath for just a few seconds. He then breathes normally, through the nose, for 2 minutes or a bit longer. He then repeats this many times over.

If you can determine the pace at which your child normally walks to the bus, you can then translate the duration of a breath hold and a 2–minute break in between into an appropriate number of steps. This is an easy way for the child to keep track of his progress without having to rely on a clock. For example, a child can do a breath hold for 5 steps, then breathe normally for 160 steps, then take 5 steps without breathing again, and then repeat the cycle.

Breath holds should be slightly challenging, and yet should not cause any signs of hyperventilation. If they do, they are too long and should be modified right away.

Remember that breath holds should be done ONLY after exhalation, NOT after inhalation.

I recommend doing this exercise for 5 to 30 minutes. Do not exceed 30 minutes.

23. Simple Jumps

Have the child do a breath hold after an exhalation by blocking his nose with his fingers. Then, with the breath held, ask him to jump energetically once or a few times. Make sure the child's mouth is closed while jumping. Afterwards, he should resume normal nasal breathing.

Next, have the child walk around a room or dance slowly for two minutes, continuing to breathe normally and calmly.

Then repeat the same number of jumps, followed by more walking.

This exercise could be done periodically throughout the day. It can come in handy if, for example, Mom is making dinner and can't fully engage with the child. She can just ask him do a few jumps, and supervise minimally, making sure the child doesn't show signs of hyperventilation.

These exercises could be done informally or as a part of a formal session.

Duration: 5 to 15 minutes.

---

24. Three-Fold Jumps

This is one of the most important exercises for kids. It can be used as a primary breathing improvement exercise.

There are three parts to each set: jumping, running in place, and walking.

~ Jumping:

Have the child do a breath hold by blocking his nose with his fingers after an exhalation and then, with the breath still held, have him jump as many times as he can. (Start with one jump when first introducing this exercise or when a child's Control Pause is very low.) Make sure the child's mouth remains closed throughout.

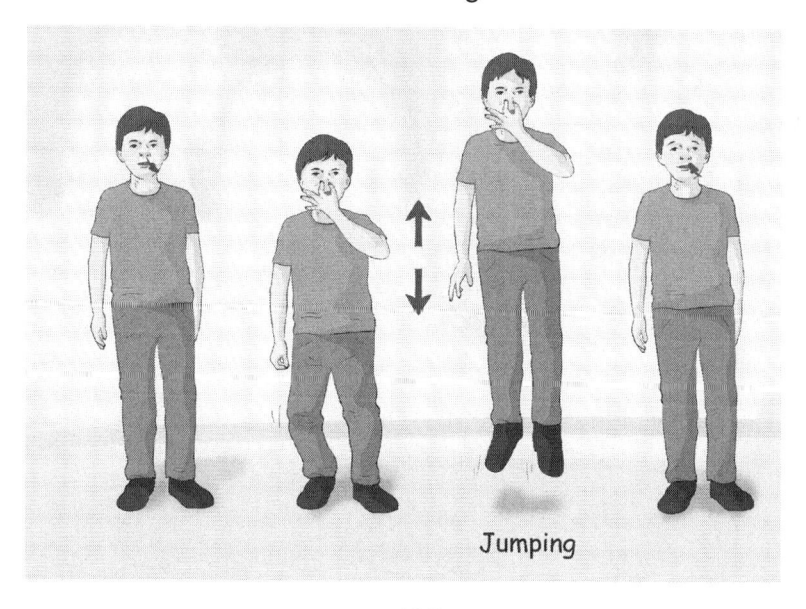

Jumping

This exercise should not trigger any signs of hyperventilation. If it does, reduce the number of jumps. The duration is determined by the number of jumps a child is capable of doing.

~ Running:

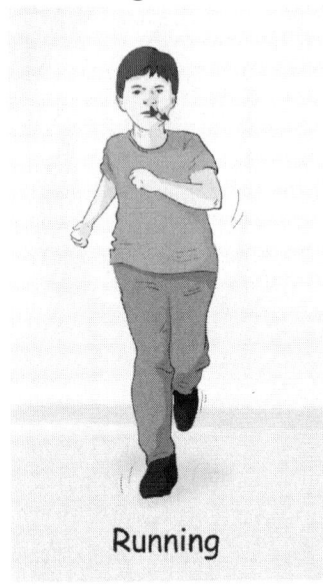

Following the last jump in a series, the child should release his nose and inhale through the nose. This first inhalation can sometimes be forceful and loud. To avoid this, explain how to divide one long inhalation into a series of smaller ones—inhaling rapidly, with several short pauses and without exhaling, similar to a dog sniffing. As soon as the child resumes breathing, he should start running as intensely as he can. He can run in place. If this exercise is done outside, don't let the child leave your sight because you will need to observe his breathing, especially at the beginning. As always, make sure he's not breathing through his mouth.

During this period of intense running, the child should breathe only through his nose and inhale as lightly as possible. Tell your child to try and breathe a little less than his body wants. This period of strenuous running should last for a maximum of 1 minute. However, at the beginning, many children find it impossible to do this part of the exercise for a full minute. If you push a child to do a whole minute, he will hyperventilate. Always practice a gentle approach! Have him run for 5 to 10 seconds at first. If he can do this without hyperventilating, then increase this part of the exercise to 20 seconds, then a bit longer, gradually building it up to a full minute. For some children with enlarged adenoids it can take a month or more to run for a minute while breathing only through the nose.

~ Walking:

Next, ask your child to walk around the room calmly or dance around slowly. This time is used to give the breathing a break from the stress of the two previous phases. During this phase, the child should breathe through his nose, but without attempting to modify his breathing.

Make sure the child doesn't talk during the walking section.

This last phase should last about 5 minutes. However, if a child is breathing heavily, he should walk calmly until his breathing quiets down.

This three-fold set can be done as a complete exercise. For best results, I recommend doing three sets of this exercise in a row every day, one to three times a day. It is great for the child to do this three-fold exercise every morning before breakfast. Hyperventilation is usually strongest in the morning, so it is essential to stop or reduce it right away. If you don't, your child will continue hyperventilating throughout the day, which will cause symptoms and contribute to further development of asthmatic symptoms.

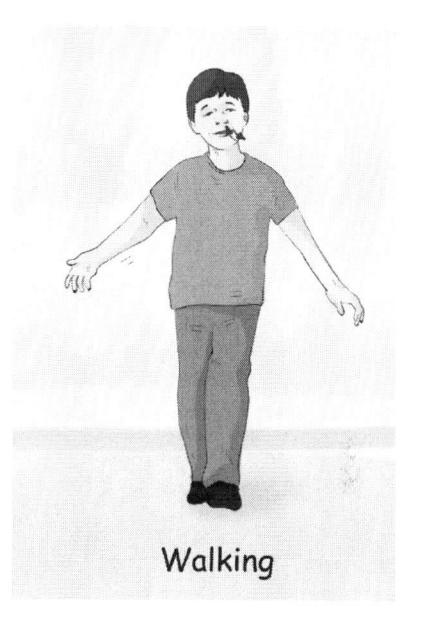

Walking

If your child is doing three sets, the number of jumps for the second and third sets should be reduced by one jump each time, to make each subsequent set a bit easier. For example, if the maximum number of jumps the child can do is five, then the first set will be five jumps, the second, four jumps, and the third, three jumps. As the child's breathing improves over time, the initial number of jumps will increase.

Please note that this exercise needs to be strictly regulated by the strength of a child's breathing, not by the strength of his body. The body of a child with enlarged adenoids might be capable of doing a hundred jumps and running for several minutes. However, his breathing capacity might allow for only two jumps and a fifteen-second run before hyperventilation sets in. Be aware of your child's breathing, and teach him to be mindful of his limitations! If these limitations are ignored, this exercise will have a negative effect, and hyperventilation and symptoms triggered by it will only get worse.

Keep in mind that this is a powerful exercise and should be treated with caution.

This is one of the most important and most effective exercises for kids. It can be used as a main breathing improvement exercise.

This exercise is always used as a part of a formal session at first, but can be used informally once a child learns how to do it during his formal sessions.

Duration: 5 to 20 minutes.

III. Breathing Exercises for Relaxation

Hyperventilation is reduced when a person is relaxed. Therefore, relaxation is an effective way to tame over-breathing.

Unfortunately, most kids have little space in their lives to relax. Their daily schedules are often filled with one activity after another—school, chorus, hockey, birthday parties, dance lessons, math tutoring, etc. It can become close to a full-time job for a parent to coordinate all these activities. The old days when children used to spend hours daydreaming or creating fantasy worlds with their friends are over for many kids today. The achievement-oriented lifestyle, often imposed on a child from a very young age, creates enormous stress and triggers over-breathing.

To maintain mental balance, kids should be allowed to spend time in their inner world. Being in an interior space counterbalances the stresses of the outside world and fosters calmness. We need to create opportunities for children to spend time in their inner world because it aids healthy breathing and overall health.

I recommend starting a session of formal breathing exercises with 5 to 10 minutes of relaxation. A child does not need to relax before every session, but should do it often.

25. Imagine

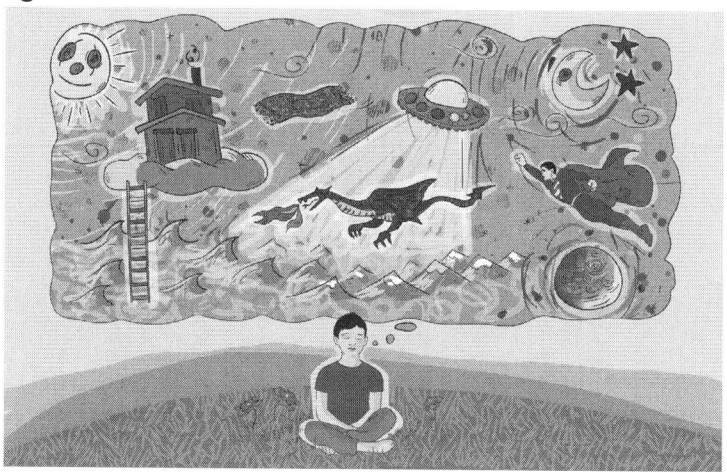

Have your child close his eyes and gently roll them upward as if he's watching a movie on a screen above his head (having the eyes in this position reduces breathing). Ask him to imagine some-thing he really likes on the screen, such as his favorite animal, brother or sister, best friend, favorite car, or a beautiful princess. Have him look at every detail of the image.

For example, ask:

"Can you see the dog's tail? Is it long or short? Is it wagging? What color is it?"

"Can you see the dog's eyes? Are they closed or open? What color are the dog's eyes? Are they happy or sad?"

After helping your child establish a mental image, start imagining with him. Ask your child to imagine the dog flying through the sky, having a great time racing around the clouds, over rainbows, etc. Have the child picture himself in the sky with his dog, flying together and meeting all kinds of imaginary beings. Suggest that he listen to the clouds and rainbows talking to him or his dog. The point is that the child exercises his imagination, experiences the freedom and joy of the inner world where the stresses of the outside world do not exist. Enjoy this mental vacation together!

This exercise is always beneficial, but especially so when the child is a bit tired, like right before bedtime. This is a fun exercise and cannot be overdone.

26. I am Not a Robot

In today's world, there is a lot of structure and restriction in kids' lives. There is less time for free play outdoors than there was a generation ago, and it is now considered normal for kids to spend hours in one position, barely moving at all while doing their homework, or for them to have their eyes locked on a computer screen. Even when children are physically active, their movements are often dictated by instructions from their coach, dance teacher, teammates, etc. If you analyze all the movements a child goes through each day, most likely you will find that it is a chain of repeated, organized "robot-like" movements devoid of improvisation and spontaneity.

The purpose of this exercise is to allow a child to move in spontaneous funny, offbeat and unpredictable ways. A child was asked to imagine a drunken person who makes all kinds of erratic and perhaps comical movements. Next, they were asked to impersonate a drunken person. Children love this exercise but—no surprise—parents would often find it "socially unacceptable." To be diplomatic, I renamed this exercise "I am not a Robot!" The essence of this relaxation exercise remains the same: to let a child's body choose how it wants to move for once, instead of following his mind, an adult's guidelines, or social norms.

This is a great informal exercise. It can also be done at the beginning of a formal session to help the child relax. Duration: 5 to 10 minutes.

27. Heating Pad

Hyperventilation can also be reduced by physically relaxing the muscles, especially muscles in the chest. A heating pad can help relax chest muscles. When your child is watching TV or involved in any other quiet activity, offer him a warm heating pad or hot water bottle to put on his chest or the area in between the two sides of the rib cage, which is where the diaphragm is (the most important muscle for breathing). Watch to see if the signs of hyperventilation—such as heavy or loud breathing or wheezing—subside.

Sometimes, the same effect can be achieved by taking a hot shower or sitting in front of a heater or a fire. The bright orange colors of a fire create an additional positive color-therapy effect for children suffering from over-breathing.

This should be done informally. Duration: 15 minutes or more.

28. Tense Up

This exercise helps relax the upper body and increase a child's understanding about sensations created through relaxation.

Ask your child to make his face as tense as possible, so that it is a tight, wrinkled cringe. Have him hold this expression for a few seconds, and then have him relax his face. Repeat three times.

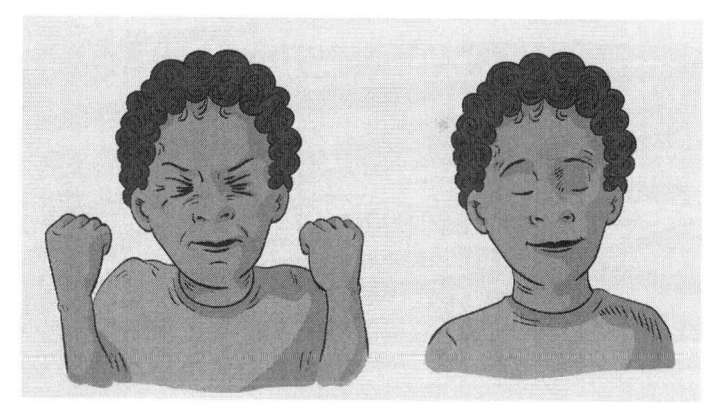

Have him do the same thing in the throat and shoulders. Repeat three times.

Have him do the same thing in the chest area. Repeat three times.

At the end of the exercise, ask your child how the different areas of his body felt when he relaxed them. Give him plenty of time to analyze and express his feelings. Make sure he understands the difference between tension and relaxation. In the future, if you want your child to relax, you can use his memory of this exercise as a reference point.

This is a great informal exercise, which can also be done at the beginning of a formal session to help the child relax. Duration: 5 to 10 minutes.

IV. Breathing Exercises to Stop Symptoms

29. Nodding

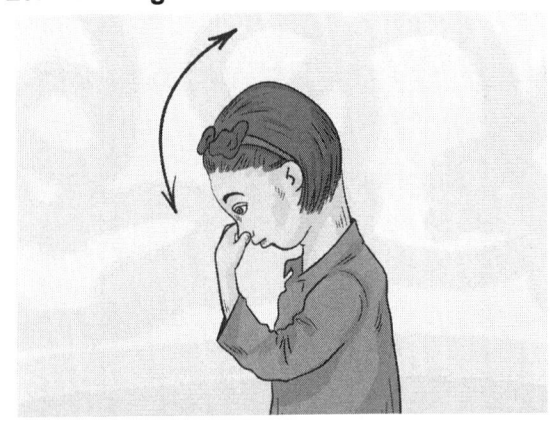

Usually, children are trained to clear their sinuses by blowing into a tissue. This process is accompanied by forceful inhalation and exhalation, which often results in a loss of carbon dioxide, promotes over-breathing and boosts symptoms.

Luckily, there is a way to clear mucus from the sinuses that does not cause any damage. Instruct your child to do the following.

Take one gentle breath: a moderate inhalation followed by a moderate exhalation. Make sure your mouth is closed. Then, pinch your nose while doing a breath hold, and start nodding your head up and down. Do it one, two or three times. Rest a little and then repeat.

This exercise is often more successful, and more of a game, if the child jumps up and down, synchronizing jumps with the nodding of his head.

30. The Breathing Guru

This exercise is not easy. It requires awareness and patience and not every child (or even adult) is able to do it!

Sit quietly and allow the body and the mind to rest. Make sure your mouth is closed and bring your awareness to the passage of air through your nose. Notice how much air your nose is allowing to pass through without any effort on your part. Relax into slow, gentle breathing.

The body is intelligent and knows exactly how much air it needs. The mind is in the habit of overriding it. If you breathe exactly as much air as your nose allows, you will significantly reduce your air intake, reducing hyperventilation. The symptoms (stuffy or runny nose, which arises as a defense mechanism against over-breathing) will decrease. If this exercise is done correctly, it is very effective. It will stop a runny nose within about 10 minutes.

The nose is probably the most underappreciated organ in the entire body. Yet, it is one of the most important ones, since its function is to condition air for our consumption and to regulate our air intake. This process determines the level of CO_2 in our lungs, which Dr. Buteyko called the main regulator for all functions of the body. Our health greatly depends on the nose. I call the nose "The Breathing Guru." There is no Breathing Normalization expert who can determine precisely how much air you need at each specific moment, but your nose can! While doing this exercise, take time to acknowledge the important role of this organ. You may want to say "thank you" to your nose to compensate for all the times you were irritated by your nose's attempts to protect your body from hyperventilation. Please explain the nose's importance and function to your child. When a child understands the function of his nose, he becomes much more successful in normalizing his breathing.

31. Coughing

Coughing is another activity that can easily result in a loss of carbon dioxide, thus promoting hyperventilation and strengthening symptoms. Typically, we cough to expel mucus from the throat, which may be necessary, but can be done in a way that doesn't cause problems.

Make sure your mouth is closed, making a gentle coughing sound three times. After that, pinch your nostrils and do a breath-hold for 1 to 3 seconds. Finally, open your nose and inhale through it in a measured way.

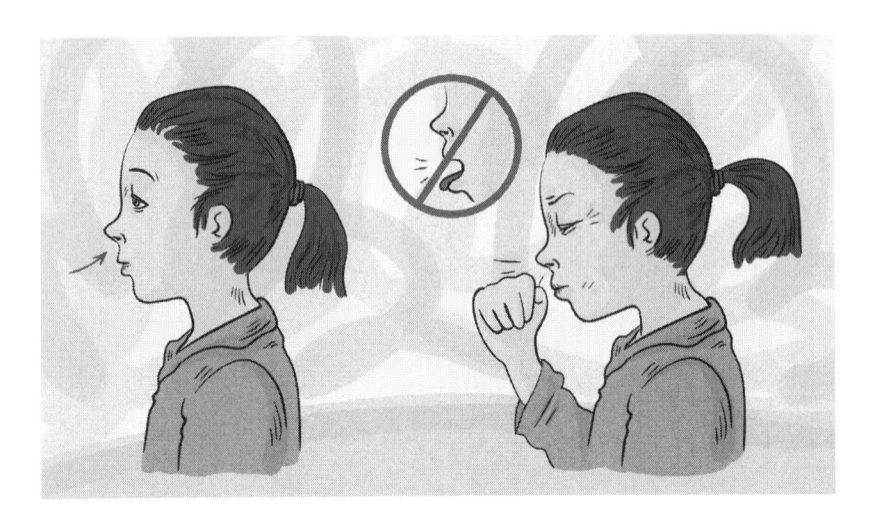

Section 6:
The Living Miracle

Part 1: Testimonials by People Who Tamed Asthma

Breathing Center has a collection of countless stories of students who greatly reduced or stopped their asthma symptoms after applying Buteyko Breathing Normalization. It was a difficult task to choose testimonials for presenting them in this book. Eventually, it was decided to choose not necessarily the strongest but a more diverse selection. Enjoy!

1. Ann Chris Warren
Kingston, NY, 2016

Before I started the Breathing Normalization Method I was living a life dependent on a rescue inhaler. I had asthma and serious sinus problems, including chronic sinusitis and stuffy nose. My asthma was mostly allergy induced and since I was allergic to everything, everything triggered an asthma attack; outdoor allergens, indoor allergens, you name it and I would have a reaction to it. One spring/summer my doctor actually advised that I refrain from spending any amount of time outside. I was on daily medications, but since my asthma was brought on by allergic triggers and I had so many, my asthma was extremely difficult to control. My doctor eventually suggested I use my rescue inhaler preventively, so when I was going to be around allergens or going to exercise, I would use it prior to that activity to prevent an asthma attack. Well, since everything was a trigger I ended up using my rescue inhaler multiple times a day, well over what the average usage should be. As a result my body became very dependent on the rescue inhaler in order to take a breath. I couldn't even take a quick jaunt from my house to the car and back without needing to use the rescue inhaler.

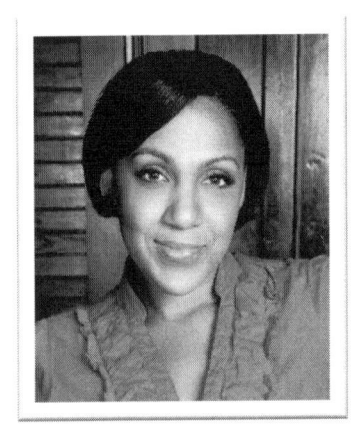

When I stumbled upon Buteyko and the Breathing Normalization Method, I was extremely skeptical. I thought there is no way this method can do all it claims to do. But Sasha and Thomas were so kind and generously gifted me the Buteyko Method CD and book to try some of the basics on my own, confident that this method would help me. They were right! It more than helped me, it changed my life. Within a very short period of time, a couple of days actually, after I started implementing the very basic first steps I could feel a difference. I took the full course with Sasha, and within the first couple of weeks my symptoms had reduced greatly and I was using my rescue inhaler a lot less. I wanted to really put the method to the test so I tried not using my rescue inhaler for a day and found that I didn't' need it. After that day I never needed to use it again.

Now, four years later, I still do not even own a rescue inhaler. This is not to say I haven't gotten sick; the method doesn't make you immune to life and immortal, but if you've applied it correctly it does change what "sick" means. In four years I have not taken a single sick day from work. In the past, getting sick always meant a trip to the doctor followed by weeks of recovery. Asthma attacks, sinus infection, bronchitis, strep throat and tonsillitis—these were extremely common for me, and I would battle one or all of them multiple times a year. Not to mention being on allergy and asthma medicine year round to combat the daily stuffy nose and breathing difficulties I had. Now, sick means feeling a little under the weather, occasional runny nose, and just feeling a bit run down. Usually this is brought on by overworking myself, and a little extra rest mixed with some thoughtful Breathing Normalization exercises, and I am good as new in a couple days. No trips to the doctor, no suffocation attacks, no harsh medications. I feel so liberated and free.

The most valuable gift I've received from applying Breathing Normalization is having a positive healthy relationship with my breathing instead of fearing it. I feared my breathing before. I feared being in a situation that would make me go into a suffocation attack. Now I don't have that fear anymore. There's a sense of freedom that goes with learning the method, knowing that you are in control of your

Part 1: Testimonials By People Who Tamed Asthma

breathing and health and are armed with the knowledge and tools to gain control should symptoms try to come. You become very aware of your breathing until it becomes second nature, then you don't even have to think about it doing things correctly, you just do it automatically. That's when you know you successfully retrained your breathing and corrected your breathing patterns. That sense of freedom is an amazing feeling.

⇉ ———— ⇇

2. Larry Arem
Merion Station, PA

Part 1, written in 2010:

I am happy to report that at my most recent check-up my pulmonologist reported that my pulmonary function tests registered the best scores since I was diagnosed with asthma, even though I am no longer taking any medication.

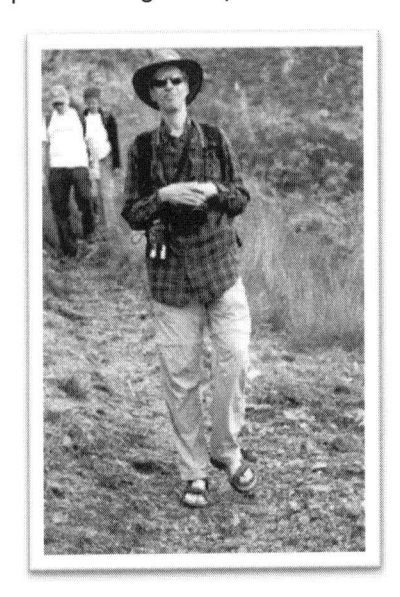

By way of background, I had trouble breathing through my nose for as long as I can remember and had been told by many doctors over a 40-year period that my turbinates were enlarged, blocking my nasal passages. At around age 50, I started intensive cycling training, always breathing through my mouth. Around age 54, I developed a milk protein sensitivity (not lactose intolerance, nor allergy) and at 58 asthma. On one long bike ride in August 2008, my coughing was so intense I had to end the ride after 90 miles. Albuterol only made the coughing worse. That is when I consulted a pulmonologist who told me my lungs were at 50% capacity, inflamed and "angry." Eventually, I wound up using a cocktail of meds via a nebulizer for a month followed by Symbicort, two puffs twice a day to control the asthma. Less drastic medicines did not stop the cough.

Then in November 2009, I read about the Buteyko Method in the *New York Times* and called Breathing Center. In late November, I began to self-treat using Buteyko ideas, and then I started individual Breathing Normalization training with Thomas Fredricksen when his schedule permitted in early December.

Breathing through my nose and doing 'less-breathing exercises' led to a clear nose. The turbinates are normal. By Christmas 2009, I was off Symbicort and only taking a steroid, at much lower dosages. It took another five or six weeks to taper off of that. I continue to do Buteyko exercises and have worked them into my daily routine. I keep my meds handy, but have not taken any for almost two months now. I tried some cheese recently and found that my reaction was minimal, almost unnoticed. I have not gone back to dairy, instead mostly following the Buteyko vegan recommendation. But I no longer live in dread of a restaurant mistake. I suspect that the benefits of breathing through my nose will extend beyond asthma control and elimination of digestive problems. Make no mistake, I still have asthma. Occasionally, I will have a cough, tight chest or some phlegm (although these happen less frequently as time passes). But these symptoms can be quickly eliminated with breathing relaxation techniques. Obviously this is not all psychological since nasal blockage is gone and objective lung function tests are normal and better than when I was on powerful medications.

I had to cut back on intense exercise during this period and am only now gradually ramping up my efforts. But I can perform today with calm breathing at levels that seemed impossible a month ago. Anyone with breathing problems short-change themselves by not giving the Breathing Normalization Method a try.

Part 2, written in 2016:
I have been asthma free since adopting the Breathing Normalization Method. For many years now I have been able to ride any bike course my legs can handle, calmly breathing through my nose. My legs will

always give out before I am too short of breath, no matter how hard the course. My rides have included New Zealand's south island, where I was the only 40+ year old rider in my group to climb three mountain passes without walking. Similarly, I easily can do a time trial breathing through my nose. I find that I get fewer colds and that their severity and duration are reduced since I have been breathing through my nose. I also no longer experience reflux and do not have dairy issues (although I still try to avoid dairy anyway). Buteyko Breathing Normalization has been a life changer for me.

3. Mike Gosselin
Ivoryton, Connecticut

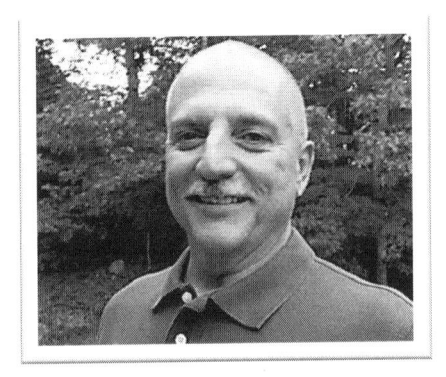

Part 1, written in 2009:

It all started when I was ten years old and came down with pneumonia. After my recovery, I started getting asthma attacks whenever I went out to play with the other kids. The doctors said I developed severe allergies, needed allergy shots and an awful tasting liquid medication. The treatment helped but did not stop it. I would still get severe attacks, just less frequently.

As the years went by the doctors said that I would grow out of it as I got older. It eased up slightly until 1985 when I ended up in the hospital with a life threatening asthma attack. I spent three days there, was given more medication and told that an attack this severe could happen again at any time. I continued using the medication and staying away from the triggers. In 2006, I came down with pneumonia again, but this time it was worse. I spent one month on steroid inhalers and Prednisone. I was told I needed to stay on steroids the rest of my life. With this treatment I started to develop stomach problems, which meant I needed another medication.

After three more years of frustration I decided to look into alternative medicine. I found the Breathing Center on the Internet and read the entire website. I could not believe that I have been hyperventilating all these years. I called Thomas Fredricksen, and after talking with him, I knew he could help me. The theory of the Buteyko Method made sense.

I met him in person and had my first session at Woodstock, NY. It was fantastic! Since then, my sessions have been on Skype, which works great. Within four days of doing the formal exercises and monitoring my breathing I reduced my medication by 75%. I'm at day 32 and on NO medication at all! I still can't believe it's true and cannot remember when I have felt this good. I still have a way to go and I'm staying focused. The best part is I have control over asthma, which has controlled me for 40 years.

Thomas, thank you for this wonderful education. You have become a true friend for life.

Part 2, written in 2010:
It has been over a year now since I started applying the Breathing Normalization Method. Before I began the method I was living on a rescue inhaler. I had no choice because my stomach would not tolerate the steroids prescribed to me. A shot of the inhaler would take away my symptoms for a few hours until I needed more. Each time I would think about the negative long-term effects the medication would have on my health. I remember the most frequent side effect was blurred side vision, which would result in migraine headaches.

With each Breathing Normalization session, I listened and learned to all that Thomas had taught me. My mind was like a sponge, absorbing each and every word. I quickly realized that this was not a quick fix but a lifelong education where I was given the tools to heal my body naturally without drugs. It was now my responsibility to insert this education into my daily life.

In the beginning I had to make time in my day to fit in formal breathing exercises. I kept in mind that my health was more important than anything else. Having good discipline paid off quickly, as I was feeling much better within each week. This gave me more motivation each day, as I needed my rescue inhaler less and less. I was on the road to success.

I've learned to reduce my breathing naturally without really thinking about it throughout the day. Stress and anxiety no longer have the negative effects on my breathing as they used to. More exercise and a better diet have also helped me feel better in many ways. I sleep less but feel much more rested in the morning and have more energy throughout the day. I recover from intense exercise or a day of yard work very quickly and do not wake up with body aches in the morning.

Oh, I almost forgot. I am no longer on any medications or suffering from asthma attacks.

Part 3, written in 2013:
Hello, Sasha,

I haven't been in touch with you for quite some time now and I've been wanting to give you and Thomas an update on how I have been doing. But first I would like to say that unfortunately my job has kept me from attending the continuing education seminars on Saturdays, and it has become quite stressful due to a lack of help. The good news is that I don't let that stress affect my breathing anymore.

It's hard to believe that I'm going on my fourth year now since I had asthma. As a matter of fact, I haven't been sick in over three years! A few times over the years I have felt what I would call the beginnings of a sore throat. Immediately I will start doing more breath holds, as many as I can throughout the day, and the soreness always goes away. Last year everyone in my office got sick except me. Back when I was still asthmatic I didn't have a chance. I'd get shortness of breath, and intense mucus would build up in my lungs.

The article you wrote the other day about nose breathing is so true. That is one of the tools I learned from you and Thomas and is the first step to good health. It's unbelievable how powerful our noses are and the amount of germs they keep out of our lungs. And allergies, forget it, they don't exist in my life anymore! I can't remember the last time I had a sneezing attack. I'm sure it was at least four years ago. Thanks to you and Thomas I am feeling better than ever, and I am free of any medication.

Part 4, written in 2016:
Hello Sasha, I would like to give you an update on my health. If I had to use one word I would say that it is Great! I was sitting the other day out on my deck thinking of how long that I had suffered with asthma. It does not seem like it was forty years. I also can't believe that I have not had an asthma attack since I learned the Buteyko Method seven years ago. I have more energy, and I am able to walk, run or split firewood without the worry of an asthma attack. The best part is that the cold winter air no longer bothers me nor do the spring allergies. Once again I cannot thank you and Thomas enough.

---

4. Cole Harris
California 2013

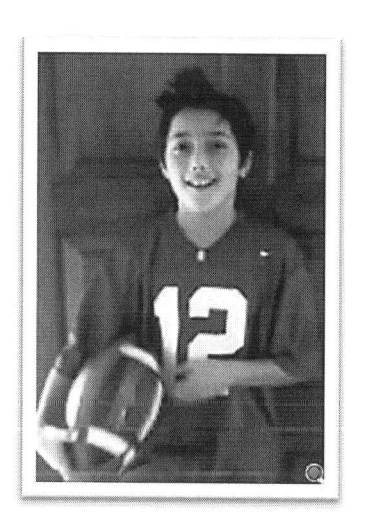

Hi, I am Cole Harris. I am twelve years old. And this is my story. I was eight and my family went on vacation, and on the last part of this trip, I suddenly was not able to breathe. I was taken to hospital and doctors said that I had asthma. And for the next two years after that, by the time I was 10, I was in an emergency room once a week with asthma attacks. And this was not going to end. I was on five meds and I was really scared. And then, I learned about the Breathing Center. I was coached by Mike, by Skype, and he told me that I should tape my mouth at night, so I can breathe through my nose. Yes, breathe through my nose! And do a few exercises. So, thank you Mike, and thank you Breathing Center that I don't have asthma attacks anymore.

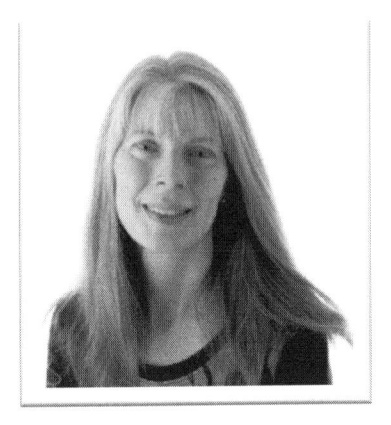

5. Monique De Leng
Holland, 2016

I am Monique De Leng, and I live in the Netherlands. I'm a Naturopath, and I want to tell you about my journey on the path of Breathing Normalization.

Let me tell you first how it all started. When I was born, I was not able to breathe well and was immediately taken to the hospital. I spent a lot of my childhood in hospitals. I often had bronchitis, strep throat, tonsillitis, adenoiditis, and I had pneumonia several times. Over the years, the ENT surgeon performed three tonsillectomies and two adenoidectomies. As I had been seriously ill several times, the pediatrician told my mother that he thought I would die before the age of seven. Yet, if I was able to reach that age, he predicted that things would get better for me. My mother made sure to follow his advice to keep me warm at all times: she dressed me with woolen clothes, gave me warm milk and hot porridge.

Just before turning seven years old, I got severe double pneumonia and spent several weeks in the hospital. I was lucky to survive. We then moved from a big city with air pollution to a small country village because my parents thought that it would be better for my breathing. Things did improve a little bit, but I still was ill often. I missed a great deal of school; I couldn't even play outside and missed many other activities healthy children could do.

After a few years, it was a time for me to start high school. A daily hour ride on a bicycle was required to get to school. Obviously, I would not be able to do this year round considering the weather in Holland. So, we moved to another town with a high school nearby. A few months later, after several occurrences of pharyngitis and bronchitis, my tonsils were removed for the third time. During this time, I had to take a lot of antibiotics.

When I became a young adult, I had a cat, which oddly enough also suffered from chronic asthmatic bronchitis. Since the cat did not react positively to conventional medicine, the veterinarian advised homeopathy. To my surprise, it gave her some relieve. This became my inspiration to study naturopathic medicine. I studied a lot, and I tried many kinds of alternatives modalities for myself. Instead of getting better, the coughing worsened; my nose was constantly blocked; my tonsillitis came back as did sinusitis, otitis, and bronchitis. I remember waking up when my husband saying to me: "You need to see a doctor today; your coughing got worse last night!" At that time I used a rescue inhaler, a preventative inhaler, auto-immunization therapy for multiple allergies, a corticoid spray for the nose, and Singulair pills for my breathing. I often needed Codeinefosfaat as well. Yet I was still ill! The doctor auscultated my lungs and said: "I am not sure if it is pneumonia but let's be on the safe side, because tomorrow is Christmas, we better get you on antibiotics now." I could not believe that it was all happening again!

I am so glad that one day, while browsing the Internet, I found out about Dr. Buteyko and his discovery. I thought, "I should try it." First, I attended a Buteyko workshop here, in the Netherlands, and then I attended a group course. Nevertheless, my health issues remained. It wasn't until 2011, when after taking the online Breathing Normalization training at BreathingCenter.com, I was able to say that my asthma was gone (or perhaps, it would be wiser to say that my asthma went to remission).

Anyway, now I am free of all medication and breathing trouble. It's great! I haven't been ill for... I don't even know how long. I haven't had a cold, and when you're asthmatic, you know what it means to have a cold. It doesn't mean you have a cold like somebody else for a few days or a week; you'll be ill for six weeks because you'll be suffering from bronchitis and other asthmatic symptoms. You'll need antibiotics, a rescue inhaler, and the whole painful circle will begin again. Instead, I enjoy not having asthma, not catching colds, not suffering from bronchitis, not having a congested nose. Breathing Normalization is fantastic!

6. David Wiebe
Woodstock, NY

Part 1, written in 2009:
Since I was ten years old, I suffered from asthma, a disease Western medicine considers incurable.

Most of the time my symptoms were under control until I developed an eye condition, macular degeneration, which in 2009 was rapidly advancing.

My retinal specialist insisted that I stop using steroids because they were exacerbating this condition. Through further research I discovered that steroid-based medication, while controlling my asthma was slowly and steadily destroying my vision. If I was going to keep my eyesight I had to quit my steroid medication. So I did, and as a result, my asthma became completely out of control! My asthma attacks became frighteningly strong, and I was frequently taken to the emergency room. To save my life, I started taking strong steroids again; however, I was about to lose my vision and my work together with it.

Through an acquaintance, I stumbled onto information about Dr. Buteyko. To my surprise I discovered the representation of Clinica Buteyko Moscow in my hometown—Woodstock, New York. Thomas Fredricksen, the Breathing Normalization Specialist in the Buteyko Center USA (later, the Breathing Center) admitted me into their program, and I got started on my path to tame my asthma.

Dr. Buteyko's approach offers a way of measuring progress, which is called the "Control Pause." It indicates one's ability to breathe in a healthful way and is designated by a numerical benchmark. When I arrived to the Breathing Center, my Control Pause was extremely low, but in two weeks it has increased five times over my initial number. As I gradually learn new techniques, I notice a distinct improvement in my daily and nightly breathing, as well as a reduced need for my medication. When I first started, I had to use my rescue inhaler from 8 to 20 times in a 24-hour period, when just in a couple of weeks, I needed it about once during the same time period. At this point, I have already improved well beyond anything I could have imagined.

Now, at about three months since I started learning Breathing Normalization, my symptoms of asthma have receded to the point that I use a minimal amount of steroids. I don't experience constant fatigue anymore. My overall health has improved significantly and I feel tremendously better. Friends who have not seen me for some time have remarked that I even look significantly better than I did before I started my breathing training.

I am still practicing my breathing exercises and implementing the Buteyko lifestyle principles. I have gone from living in a very deteriorated state of health, always fearing the arrival of the next attack, to now living almost as if I no longer have asthma. I am much more comfortable and relaxed in my daily life and am very grateful to the Breathing Center for giving me my life back!

For me, Breathing Normalization is a heaven sent gift. I will practice the Buteyko Method for the rest of my life, now with hope for a long and healthy life.

Part 2, written in 2016:

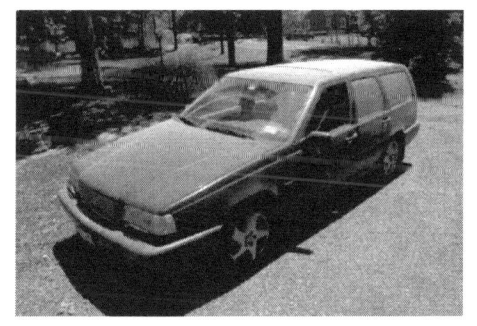

Regarding the asthma, I have been doing very well. This late spring and early summer were VERY heavy pollen seasons (see attached foto). That is my black car, all yellow with a coating of pollen on it last week. Irritants such as those allergens can make my breathing more difficult, but knock wood, I have not needed to use any Prednisone for over a year. I am still using the portable nebulizer, which administers micro doses of albuterol. But the percentage of albuterol to saline solution is .083%, so very light mixture. Most times I think of it more of a saline mist which helps loosen lung congestion to help clear the lungs.

Susan Lipkins (the wife of David Wiebe)
Woodstock, NY

Part 1, written in 2009

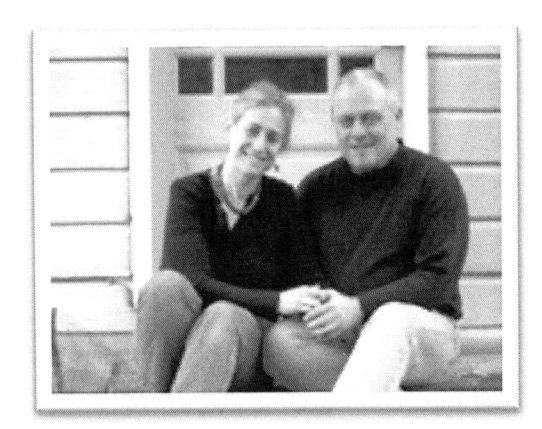

It was frightening and stressful to watch my husband suffer through his asthma attacks. I was concerned how long he could continue in this compromised state of ill health. I was praying daily for his recovery from his asthma.

I feel that my prayers were answered the day we learned about the Buteyko Method of breathing. I feel very fortunate to have the Buteyko Center USA (later, Breathing Center) located directly in our own town of Woodstock, NY, as we were prepared to travel some distance to learn this technique. Thomas Fredricksen, our instructor was understanding and supportive, not only to David, but to me—his caregiver. I was gratified to be undergoing the training of the Buteyko Method of breathing alongside David. This allowed me to help David improve his breathing and to utilize the techniques more effectively because I was also taking the training and striving to breathe less.

Thomas is an inspiring teacher, whose caring manner makes learning this method a positive, empowering experience. A side benefit to the miraculous easing of David's asthmatic symptoms, are my improved clarity of mental focus and renewed vigor. I am so grateful for the gift of health and hope you have given to us both. Thank you!

Part 2, written in 2010:
It's been about a year and a half that I have been practicing the Buteyko Method of breathing. My control pause varies between 20 and 40 seconds, depending on what I've been eating and doing, how much stress is in my life, etc. I've stopped getting colds. I have more energy than when I started doing Breathing Normalization.

I'm happy to report that my enlarged thyroid has shrunk considerably, although it is not completely gone. I have no thyroid symptoms, and I believe it will recede entirely as my Control Pause increases. It is a deep habit of mine to only breathe through my nose, and on the rare occurrence that I do inhale through my mouth, it feels so wrong—I'm shocked by it and stop immediately.

But the biggest gift of Buteyko in my life is the effect it has had on my asthmatic husband, David Wiebe. No longer do we wake up in the middle of the night with his asthma attacks. He can work in his profession of violinmaker again, and our lives do not center around his asthma. What a gift! Thank you Sasha and Thomas for giving us our lives back.

7. Breathing Center's Student New York City 2010

Dear Breathing Center,

I want to relay some happy news: I was able to run in and complete the NYC Marathon this past Sunday, November 7th. I have attached a picture of myself at the finish line with my medal (and the Breathing Center's Stop Watch) around my neck.

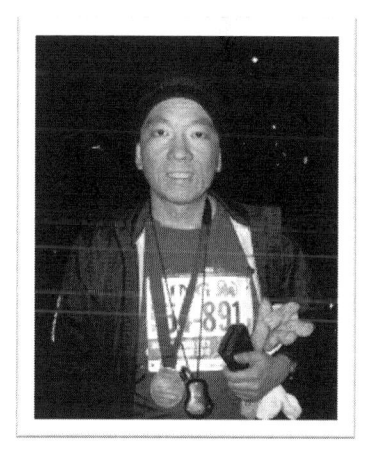

Although my time was longer than I hoped (over 6 hours), I want to say that applying the Breathing Normalization Method every day helped me to attain this accomplishment. I attended July's weekend workshop led by Thomas and Sasha. I have practiced the Buteyko breathing techniques every day since then, and my asthma has gotten significantly better. For example, my medication use has dropped to approximately one use of a preventative inhaler every 3-4 weeks and none of the rescue inhaler. Thank you for all of your help!

God Bless you, Signature of the student

8. F. R., age 15
New Paltz, NY, 2010

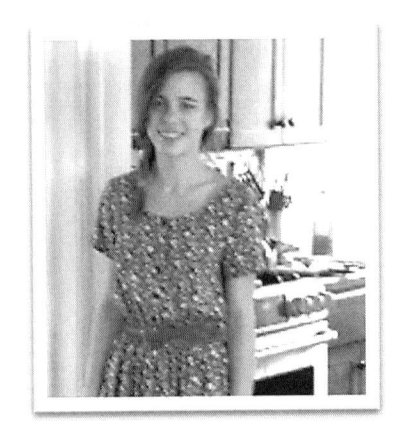

Buteyko Breathing Normalization has been a great experience. It has not only relieved me from my asthma symptoms but also enabled me to do many other things, including playing field hockey this past fall. And in the spring, I plan to play lacrosse. I first heard about Breathing Center when both my uncle and grandma sent us the article about it from *The New York Times*. We bought the CD, and I tried doing at least one exercise once a day. I was not able to make real progress however, and when my asthma became very bad over the summer my parents and I finally decided to fully apply ourselves to this method by taking a course at the Breathing Center.

When I went to my first session, I had a Control Pause of seven seconds and was having asthma attacks regularly. I had been using a rescue inhaler for my asthma since sixth grade. Since finishing the course with Sasha Yakovleva, I very rarely have any symptoms, and the two times I have some, I was able to relieve them without using my inhaler; I have not taken any medication for four months. My control pause is now twenty-three. This year I joined my school's field hockey team and I had no trouble with my asthma for the entire season. The Breathing Normalization Method has been extremely beneficial and enlightening for me.

9. Cathy Vogt
Upstate New York, 2012

During the winter 2010, I was extremely sick with asthma. I was at the point that I was not able to leave my bed to go to the bathroom without having hyperventilation and suffocation attacks. I had heard about the Breathing Center before and decided to take their program. At that time the Breathing Center's office was located in Woodstock, NY, just a few miles away from my home. Nevertheless, I was too weak to drive there, so I was very thankful for the fact that I could work with a Breathing Normalization Specialist one-on-one online without leaving my home.

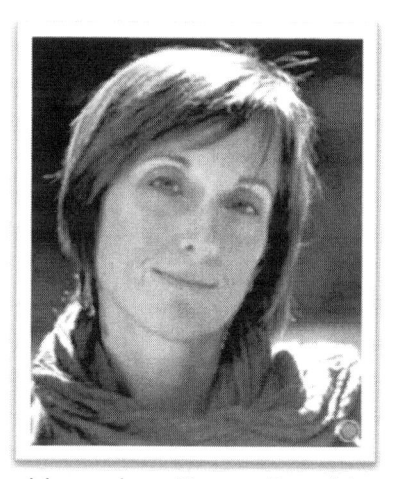

I believe I was born a hyperventilator. I was very sick even as a child. During my life I had been on many types of medication and eventually got to the point where any medication I was taking was not helping me any longer. My health was rapidly deteriorating, and I was searching for some answers—anything that would change my condition and stop my life from going downhill.

So I took the breathing training. From the moment I started working with Thomas and Sasha, I was immediately set at ease and felt very hopeful that there would be some help for my condition. And it was!

I followed exactly what I was instructed to do and within the first couple of weeks, I noticed a great deal of changes. I became able to move around without asthma attacks. Also, I was able to sleep at night when before my strong symptoms kept me awake for most of the night.

Now, two years later after learning the Breathing Normalization Method, I continually see my health improving in many small and large ways. My Control Pause keeps growing and together with it, my energy level is increasing and my health is getting stronger. I am able to enjoy outdoor activities—biking, hiking and canoeing. Last winter I was able to be outside without fear of being out of breath, when before, going into cold winter air was not an option at all. Even a thought about it would make me feel nervous!

Prior to taking the Breathing Normalization course, my asthma would stop me not only from moving but also from working. I lived in a constant fear of having an asthma attack at any moment. Now I am back to a regular life! I'm busy working, exercising, taking care of my family, and I am feeling well.

10. Charles LaBarre M.S., L.Ac., Licensed Acupuncturist
Woodstock, NY, 2009

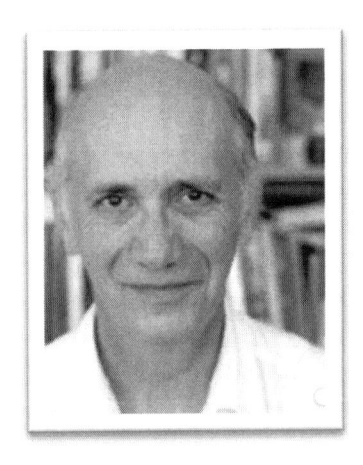

I came to the Breathing Normalization system by accident, or by fate, depending on how one sees things. My wife Doris phoned the Breathing Center after seeing a poster promoting a workshop. During the conversation, she told Thomas of my exercise-induced asthmatic condition. He then invited us to tea at the Breathing Center's lovely office. After much discussion, we both enrolled in the Breathe-less training.

I had been having progressively worse asthma symptoms whenever I would hike or go cycling. After starting Buteyko Breathing

Normalization, the very next time I went hiking my symptoms nearly vanished! Since that time, I have had no asthmatic attacks, or even hint of an attack. My hiking companions comment on how different I have been, as I used to stop frequently to "cough my head off."

In addition, the inflammation in my partially torn Achilles tendon has reduced at least 75%, and I've had far less pain and discomfort than in the last three years since it tore. It had been getting worse! A side benefit, if I may call it that, is that I have lost 5 kilos (we don't own a pounds scale) without trying to diet or change eating habits. My appetite is reduced, and I feel full much sooner and am less likely to take seconds at a meal. I believe that normalization of breathing made my metabolism more efficient, the proof being the pounds shed with no other reason evident.

Last year I was hospitalized with crippling back pain. Scans found no evident damage, so the doctors drugged me with painkillers, tranquilizers, steroids and muscle relaxers. The drugs got me out of the hospital, but left me with severe cognitive deficits that hardly began to resolve until I had been out for six months. It was then a slow incremental process of improvement, but I hadn't yet felt back to normal when we began Buteyko Breathing Normalization. Since then, I feel I have gotten back to 100% and more. My mind is clearer, and short-term memory has much improved.

It also needs to be said that this all has happened in six weeks! I'm amazed, and so grateful to Thomas and Sasha for their attention to our process. I highly recommend Breathing Normalization training to any and all who suffer with asthma and other problems.

11. Larry Thomas
West Hurley, NY, 2013

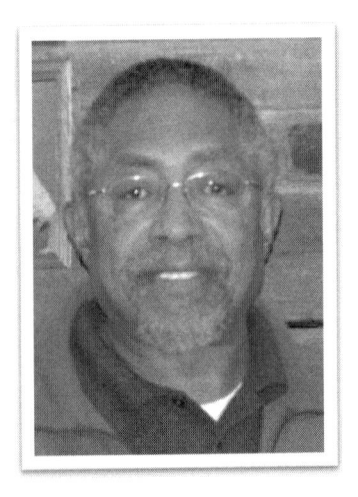

I have been suffering from asthma and allergies for 38 years. My allergies where so bad, that I've had to take shots twice a week, for almost two years. I have taken almost every drug that is available. Right now I am still taking some of them, but since I have been applying the Buteyko Breathing Normalization method I have been able to cut my medications in half!

As I learned how Breathing Normalization works, I realized that what I had been doing, for the last 30 plus years, was all wrong. I always took a deep breath through my mouth as I took my medicines. Also whenever I coughed or sneezed I took a deep breath. I always thought it would help to keep my lungs clear.

I decided to try the Breathing Normalization method because of my daughter. A friend of hers had taken the Level 1 Breathing Normalization training and had great results. I, on the other hand, had just had a bout of hyperventilation where I almost passed out. I had come to the realization that I had to do something.

It has been seven months since I started the course. My best Control Pause is 45 seconds. I know that if I keep it up, I can do so much more. The problem I see now is, when you are feeling good you think you no longer need to do the practices.

12. Kimberly Horning
Boulder, CO

Part 1, written in 2015:
Our seven-year-old daughter had her first asthma attack when she was three. After trying every supplement I could find to help her breathing difficulties (instigated by allergy, over-exertion and viruses), I turned to modern medicine. The allergy and asthma specialist prescribed asthma medicine, which worked beautifully for a month; when it lost its efficacy they gave us another drug, then another drug and finally prescribed a steroid.

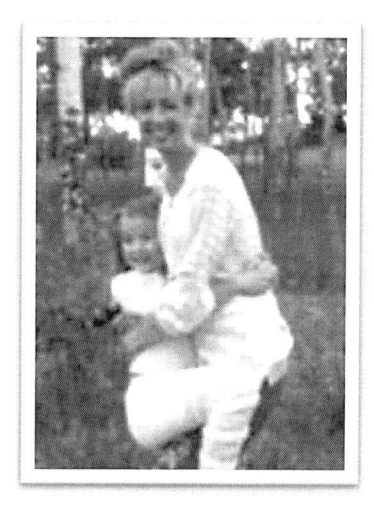

A month later, our daughter became sick with a cold, followed by another, and another, and another. Every month she was getting ill, but the last time she was sick—taking a rescue inhaler every 2-4 hours and a steroid inhalant—she said, "Mommy, I'm losing my breath walking to the bathroom or even drinking a glass of water". That's when I contacted the Breathing Center—desperate for a solution.

Bella and I Skyped with Sasha, twice a week at first and then once a week thereafter. Sasha laid the foundation for Bella to rebuild her health through very specific breathing exercises. It gives me great joy to say that my daughter no longer needs Albuterol, and she skates and jumps just as hard as I do.

Additionally, she caught a cold last weekend that lasted for three days. When a coughing fit ensued, I contacted Sasha who gave specific instructions on how to cough through her nose. In the middle of the night Bella woke up, coughing and wheezing. I gave her Sasha's instructions on how to cough through her nose and her coughing quickly subsided, her wheezing continued for minutes and then she was fast asleep.

I'm so thankful for this information and to Sasha for her dedication to improve the quality of people's lives through natural healing.

Part 2, written in 2016:
Bella is doing excellent! She is free of asthma attacks and asthma medication. I am very grateful to Sasha and Breathing Centers' support.

---

13. Diane Fitzgerald
Brooklyn, New York, 2013

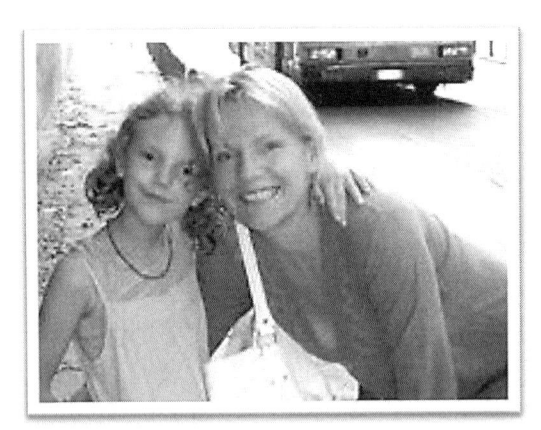

My story is one that still shocks me today when I tell it to family and friends. The day I called the Buteyko Center USA (later, Breathing Center) the summer of 2010, I was suffering from "exercise-induced" asthma that made it impossible for me to walk up a hill or a flight of stairs without wheezing. My doctor prescribed me steroids and bronchodilators that he said I would be taking the rest of my life. I was also diagnosed with a low functioning thyroid and further prescribed medication that was expected to be taken for life. I was anemic, with dangerously low iron stores and taking supplements in hopes of improving that condition. I was on a slippery slope of medical intervention that I knew was, at best, treating my symptoms, not the problem, and at worst, making me much sicker.

I knew from the first phone conversation I had with the Breathing Center that these folks were going to help. They were so confident that they could improve my condition, it was the first time I'd felt hopeful since being diagnosed. The science and logic behind their method made perfect sense to me; for reasons of stress or lifestyle, I was hyperventilating, and the imbalance of oxygen and CO2 in my body as a result of my hyperventilation was making me sick and causing my bronchial tubes to constrict in response. The constriction was, of course, my asthma.

Within a couple of days of merely beginning to implement the Buteyko Breathing Normalization Method, I felt considerably better. Within a couple of months, I stopped wheezing altogether. Six months ago, I stopped taking all of my prescribed medication and supplements, even for my thyroid and anemia. I went to the doctor recently, and my routine blood test showed that I am no longer anemic. My thyroid function is normal, and my iron stores are fine. I didn't need a doctor to confirm that I no longer suffer from asthma. Tomorrow, I am running my first road race since I was diagnosed with asthma. The staff of Breathing Center saved my life. There is no doubt in my mind.

14. Christianna Janes
Glascow, Kentucky, 2011

Seemingly at the end of a long and ever increasingly difficult struggle, I was certain my life would end soon. I was about to give up the fight completely, mainly from battle fatigue. I had to fight to breathe, fight to live, fight for understanding, (even among those that were "supposed" to understand the most). Truth be told, I was just so tired of fighting.

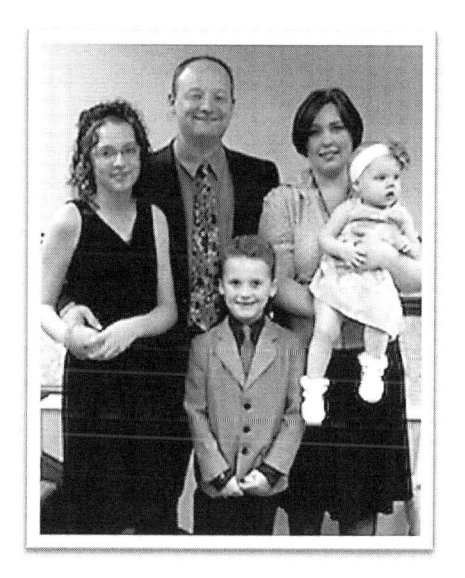

Most of the time, asthmatics are told to simply avoid our triggers and take our medications, and we, too, can live a normal life. That statement was infuriating to me because it just isn't true! Avoiding my triggers meant a lonely life, inside my own home, away from people and any scents or smells (even smoke on a person's clothing in the grocery store would send me into a weeklong asthma attack), animals, dust, the outdoors, (the list goes on and on). It meant waving goodbye to my husband and children as they had no choice but to leave me at home while they engaged in life. Taking my medications meant being on nearly every asthma drug there is and still fighting to breathe, while gaining an inordinate amount of weight due to steroids and the sedentary life I was forced into. I was trapped inside a failing vessel, and I felt that not only was I of no use to my family, but that I was also holding them back.

One night, I had been searching the internet for anything I had not yet tried when I came across Breathing Center's website. I was not overly hopeful (I'm chronically skeptical), but I filled in the Self-Test, and forgot about it. A few days later, after a particularly frustrating afternoon, I received a call from Thomas. I was surprised that the co-founder of Breathing Center was calling me personally. We talked for a while, and I cried through nearly the entire conversation. That conversation was the beginning of a profound change in my life. When we began the course, Thomas informed me that the outcome of his training would rest entirely upon me, and that it would be a commitment I would need to make to myself.

By the end of our first session, I was determined to make that commitment because for the first time, with no medication, the constriction in my chest was gone.

Later that week, I began having trouble breathing, and during a session with Thomas, we talked about it. I told him how angry I was over the things that had happened in my life, and how angry I was in general at everything. He taught me that my anger and frustration was causing much of my breathing difficulty, and that it was more important to protect my freeness of breath than it was to allow myself to become upset. I had a choice, and I needed to choose to let my anger go.

I am a better person for it, and my family has noticed greatly. For this one aspect of the training, I will remain forever grateful.

I have not used my inhalers in a month, when before, I used them several times a day. My breathing is no longer my enemy, I am MUCH calmer, my sensitivity to smells is decreasing, my energy is returning, and my allergies seem to also be easing. So, not at the end anymore, but instead at the beginning of an ever decreasingly difficult struggle, I stand eternally grateful to Thomas and Breathing Center and to those that taught my teacher, for giving me the tools to not only take back my life, but to make it even better.

15. Richard Bannister
Columbia, MD

Part 1, Written in 2010:

Until I applied Breathing Normalization, I suffered from asthma attacks, or the threat of one, since I was a small child. My condition was triggered by exercise, dust, animals, and who knows what else. For almost fifty years I took asthma medication every day. While I led a healthy lifestyle, exercising every day, eating wholesome food and trying to reduce allergens in my home, I was dependent upon pharmaceutical drugs to give me the feeling that I could breathe with comfort.

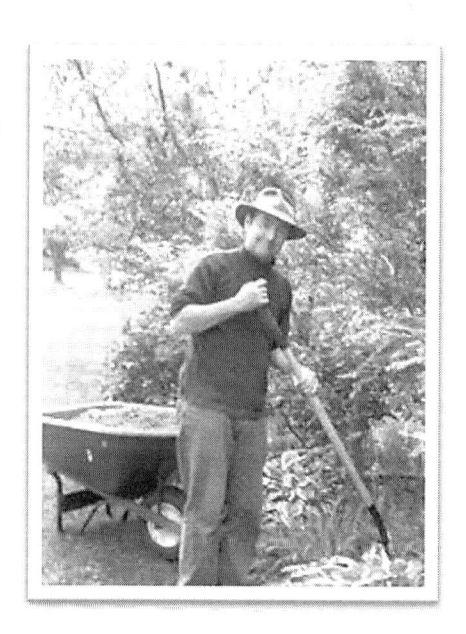

My asthma seemed well under control using medication every night, but I worried about the side effects, having read the long list that comes with each prescription. I was also tired of shelling out close to

$200 for each refill, as my insurance didn't cover it. When I came across the *New York Times* article, I thought, "What have I got to lose?" I visited the Breathing Center's website and bought the *Buteyko Breathing Exercises & Method* CD, and through diligent application of the techniques given thereon, I was able to get stop my inhaler use within a few weeks. However, my recovery felt rocky and I was intrigued as to how far this practice could be taken, so I enrolled in the Level 1 Breathing Normalization training. I'm happy to say, it has freed me from my dependence on drugs and now I enjoy having the knowledge that I need not have an asthma attack again.

But it goes beyond that. ("But wait, there's more!") I feel better in my physical being than I have in years. I now live my life in a more relaxed state; I find the time to drive more slowly and don't feel so offended by the bad habits of other drivers. I have more clarity of thought, greater concentration and a general overall improvement in health. In yoga, my body seems to be gaining elasticity at a faster pace and my muscles recover more quickly. While others around me seem to be suffering from allergies, mine have not bothered me. My guitar playing is more focused and even my singing has improved! I find I need less sleep and so have gained the time in which to do the exercises. I feel better than I have in years!

Consequently, I want to offer my thanks to my teachers, Thomas Fredricksen and Sasha Yakovleva, to their teachers Konstantin Buteyko, Ludmila Buteyko and Andrey Novozhilov, and to everyone else who has helped bring the Buteyko Breathing Normalization method into my life.

Part 2, Written in 2016:
It has been more than six years since I stopped taking medications for asthma. After a lifetime of taking drugs on a daily basis to control attacks, I remember the day I stopped as the beginning of a new kind of freedom. No more trips to the pharmacist. No more checking to see if I had an inhaler ready for "just in case" whenever I left the house. No more calls to the doctor at all, because a side effect of having done the method is that I haven't even had the flu or a serious cold since then. I was, for the first time in my life, well, and I've not missed

a day of work or play due to illness since. Actually, it's not really a side effect. It is what it is all about, this "Buteyko Method" that I practice.

I have now become a Breathing Normalization Specialist, so that I can help share this remarkable discovery and guide those who seek a holistic, gentle remedy for asthma many other conditions.

16. George Trejo, Jr
Newburgh, NY, 2012

Incredible!! That's the first word that comes to mind when reflecting on the dynamic changes that Breathing Center brought me.

Asthma plagued me when I was younger but it seemed to go away. I thought it was gone for good, until it relentlessly returned without mercy in my early 20s. I thought I'd never be able to play my saxophone again when an asthma attack hit me hours before an important performance. Attending college for music and not being able to play any wind instruments all of a sudden was obviously a huge problem. Not to mention living day-to-day depending on steroids, which had frightening side effects. My heart would race, my breathing would increase, and I often felt scared nearly to death. I often had to go to the nearest hospital's emergency room just to bring temporary relief. I was extremely fortunate to have the opportunity to attend a workshop at the Breathing Center. That wonderful two-day experience exposed me to Breathing Normalization in a comfortable group setting, while still getting my questions answered.

I then realized that their Full Training, which is a one-on-one, two-month long experience with amazing daily support and follow-up, was extremely worth the tuition. I applied what I was taught daily and progressed rapidly to a full recovery. I can't say enough about how much my life has changed for the better thanks to Sasha, Thomas, and the Breathing Center.

This experience has taken me from being an invalid to near perfect health, and I continue to get even healthier. My entire body has improved! Every aspect of my health has been positively impacted by applying the Breathing Normalization Method.

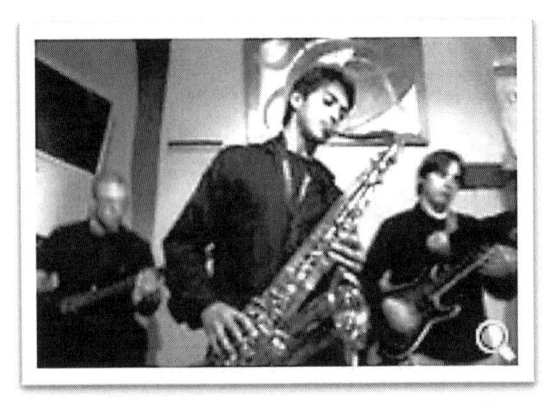

I run, I work out and most importantly to me (and my growing number of fans) I CAN PLAY THE SAX AGAIN. Whatever your personal health challenge is, find the freedom from illness that I and many others have found through the Breathing Center. It will be one of the greatest moves you've ever made.

17. Jesse Steinberg
San-Francisco, CA

Part 1, Written in 2012

I had been a prisoner of asthma for twenty-five years of my life. On top of it, I had terrible allergies, digestive issues, and extremely low energy and had experienced brain fog all the time. All these symptoms and many others were intense. I always carried a rescue inhaler, a steroid inhaler, and was rarely able to go a day without medication. I was only twenty-five years old!

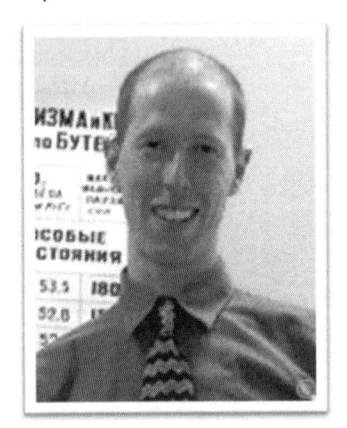

In 2009 I attended a Breathing Center's workshop where over the course of two days, Thomas and Sasha gave us a comprehensive overview of the Breathing Normalization Method. They taught the basic theory, breathing exercises and lifestyle. The workshop was a delightful experience. Thomas and Sasha are dynamic and giving teachers and their passion and depth of understanding of Dr. Buteyko's work was impressive.

Within just one week after this workshop I have already improved dramatically. With careful daily practice of the relaxation and "reduced breathing" exercises, my breathing became significantly gentler, and I did not need to use my rescue inhaler anymore. Additionally, I found myself being calmer, with greater mental clarity and more sustained physical energy. Moreover, I discovered that as I breathe better, my hereditary gastro-intestinal disorder has also improved, as has my hypoglycemia, as have my stress levels, and my posture, and my mood. Breathing was very powerful indeed!

This workshop helped me to understand my asthma and gave me confidence that with proper application of the Breathing Normalization Method I would never suffer from asthma again. It is a rare gift that Thomas and Sasha bestowed. They have given me the tools to take my healing into my own hands, and to dramatically improve my health on all fronts. Perhaps most importantly, they have empowered me to see myself as a vibrant, healthy young man, rather than a sickly person trapped by illness.

So by now I've been practicing the Breathing Normalization method for two years and eight months. It's been an incredible journey! In terms of my asthma, I stopped using all asthma medication soon after I took a workshop at the Breathing Center. I did not need it anymore. It took a number of months for my allergies to go away, but eventually, my reduced breathing made them disappear. I have no problem with my energy level anymore. I am able to run barefoot outside for many miles without having any problems. It is with great pleasure that I can say that I have come so far with my health, from someone who was very ill to someone who is healthy. I used to be the sickest person in a room, but now I often feel that I am the healthiest. Breathing Normalization not only helped me to create wellness in my life but also a sense of joy. I thank the Breathing Center for that.

Part 2, Written in 2016:
I have been practicing Buteyko Breathing Normalization for almost 7 years (since Oct 2009). It has changed everything. My life-long asthma is a distant memory. The big idea that a person's breathing state is reflected in their physiology, their mind, their connection to energy and spirituality, and their entire life is one of the most powerful teachings I have ever received.

---

18. Jill Anderson
Morristown, NJ, 2010

Part 1, written in 2010:
When my teenage son was diagnosed with asthma following severe seasonal allergies in 2009, the physician prescribed daily medication and a rescue inhaler. He said it was the only option we had. After taking his medications regularly for several months, my son still felt constant tightness in his chest and was unable to run competitively as he had prior to becoming ill. The doctor did not seem to believe that my son was still having problems.

Fortunately, Jane Brody published her *New York Times* article on the Buteyko Method a couple of months later, and we were able to attend a Breathing Normalization workshop within weeks of reading the article. It's now been nearly a year since my son and I learned Dr. Buteyko's Breathing Normalization. He is now off all medications and is the fastest runner on his high school cross-country team.

I am no longer worrying about the long-term effects and cost of the medications he was taking. Personally, for the first time in years I did not need to take any allergy medicine when all the plants were blooming this spring. The Breathing Normalization method allowed us to treat the cause of our asthma and allergy symptoms instead of simply relieving the symptoms with medication. I look forward to teaching this unique Method to others so they too can experience the benefits of breathing less.

Part 2, written in 2016:

I am proud to say that my son is a young adult living on his own who still *does not* suffer from asthma or take any medications for it. I am finding the same with my seasonal allergies. The Breathing Normalization tools continue to work for our family. We owe so much to the Breathing Center for putting us on the right path to a healthy life.

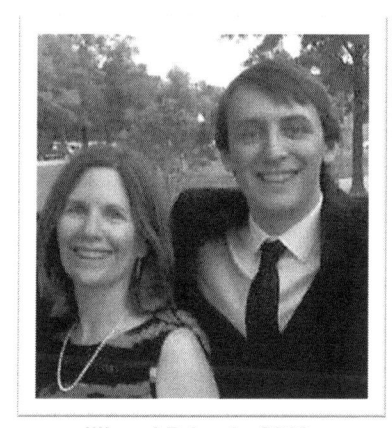

Jill and Brian in 2016

---

19. Robert Operman
Brooklyn, NY, 2014

For as long as I can remember, I've had a stuffy nose. People would say "Why don't you just blow your nose?" I would try, but nothing would come out and my nose wouldn't feel any clearer. I never understood why I had this problem, and it was extremely frustrating. When I would get colds in the winter, my nose would often close up so much that I had to breathe through my mouth for most of the day. I also would breathe through my mouth during sleep and wake up with a dry, sore throat every morning. Getting out of bed was a huge struggle because I never felt well rested.

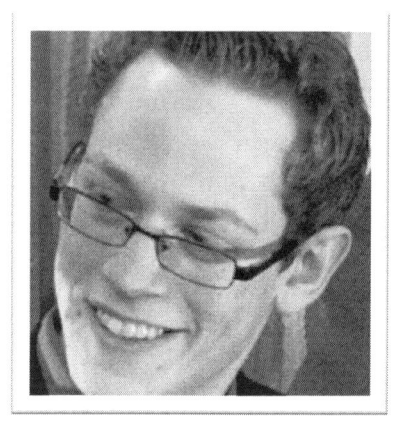

As early as high school, I suffered from daytime sleepiness and a general lack of energy. I would often fall asleep through entire class periods only to be woken up by someone nudging me because I was snoring. Again, I didn't understand why I was so tired when everyone else around me seemed to be full of energy, enjoying the physical peak of their lives.

In college I finally hit rock bottom. By the end of my freshman year I had gained 30 pounds, was developing huge red stretch marks on my chest, and I constantly felt tired, frustrated, and depressed. I also noticed that I would yawn throughout the entire day no matter how much sleep I had the night before, and I would often have the feeling that I could not take a satisfying breath, like I was not getting enough air. At this point I knew something had to change.

I read several books on nutrition, and began to incorporate a more plant-based diet. This helped me lose some weight, but did not fix all of my symptoms. I eventually decided to take more extreme dietary measures, beginning with a low-carbohydrate, anti-candida diet for about four years. I also began to exercise and do yoga. These changes improved my overall health, appearance, and energy levels, but I still felt like something was missing. I felt anxious more often than not, I could not think or communicate clearly, and I STILL had a stuffy nose a lot of the time. I felt better, but I didn't feel healthy.

As I was completing my first year of physical therapy school, I finally got tired of being on such a restrictive diet. After sticking to it religiously for four years, I didn't feel like I was getting any healthier. At that point I decided that a high-calorie, high-protein diet combined with weight training might take me to the next level in my health pursuit. I was able to pack some muscle with this combination; however, at this time my breathing issues got much worse. The feeling that I could not take a satisfying breath was preventing me from falling asleep at night. I would lay there desperately trying to yawn, because that seemed to be the only thing that would temporarily relieve the feeling of oxygen starvation I was experiencing. It was at this time that I started to research ways to naturally improve breathing, and I found Breathing Center.

I have since taken the Breathing Normalization courses levels I, II, and III. Out of all the money, time and effort I've spent in my pursuit of health, these courses have been by far the most worthwhile investment yet. After learning from Sasha and Thomas, I have experienced incredible changes in my health and my life. Now, I am very calm most of the time. My energy and mental clarity are better than they have ever been. My relationships have improved. I no longer have to breathe through my mouth. If I ever do get a stuffy nose now (which is rare), I know exactly how to clear it up completely in under a minute. I no longer have constant stiffness in my lower and upper back. Best of all, I never feel that I am starving for air. In all I feel like I have been given a second chance at life.

As my own health continues to improve, it becomes increasingly clear that my progress is limited by the health of those around me. When the people I am surrounded by are not happy and healthy, I can only progress so far with breathing exercises and lifestyle changes. In fact, all people on this earth are connected in some way or another, and a chain is only as strong as its weakest link. Therefore, I've taken up the mission to spread this incredible knowledge to as many people as possible. As a Breathing Normalization Specialist, I pass the gift of incredible health to my students, all the while becoming healthier and happier myself.

---

20. Olga Wharton
Flower Mound, TX

Part 1, Written in 2010:

Dear Jesse,

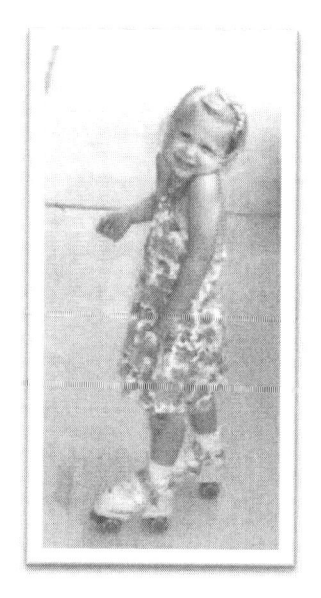

Kate, my three-year-old daughter, has been doing great, knock, knock on wood. We are still doing breathing exercises twice a day on a regular basis, and she has gotten into a habit of breathing through her nose all the time. I am very impressed with the results, as we've been having all our windows open, the pollen counts are high, everyone is coughing and sneezing, but her nose remains clear. She sleeps with open windows, plays outside, runs, jumps, and has been off medicines for 3.5 weeks now! Since her allergies have always been mild, I think that the nose breathing has really made a difference.

Her asthma has also been pretty much under control. She is still on her co-steroid inhaler twice a day, and I am just waiting for her to get a cold to see if she weathers it without a bronchodilator.

Once that happens, I'll request re-evaluation and lowering the dosage of the rescue inhaler as well. So I'm just waiting for that cold—how crazy! She hasn't had a cold for over a month now.

It really made such a huge difference to have that one Skype session with you! I am pretty sure that doing the exercises correctly is the only reason for our normal life right now. Thank you again so much!!!

Part 2, Written in 2016:
I am happy to report that Kate has been off allergy and asthma meds since 2011, since I caught her asthma early, and I implemented Breathing Normalization right after her first asthma attack happened. Her airways weren't scarred at that point, and Buteyko breathing exercises reversed the process. She's been symptom free ever since! Our pediatrician was very impressed, too, saying that a three-year old doesn't simply "outgrow" asthma by the age of four. She is ten now, and is still breathing through her nose. We don't do breathing exercises anymore, but to this day, I know that it was the books, online material, and the Skype sessions that solidified my research, and together all that contributed to her healing. I am grateful that I discovered BreathingCenter.com

and the assistance of Breathing Normalization Specialists when everyone was telling me that one can't cure asthma. I am thankful that you are bringing Dr. Buteyko's research to the public.

21. Susan Miller
Bakersfield, California, 2015

I started experiencing shortness of breath when I was 17. Since then, I had this feeling every time I was taking vitamins or pain medication. I saw many doctors who gave me various reasons for my out-of-breath feeling, but never a clear one. Not being able to understand the cause of my breathing trouble, I just learned to live with it.

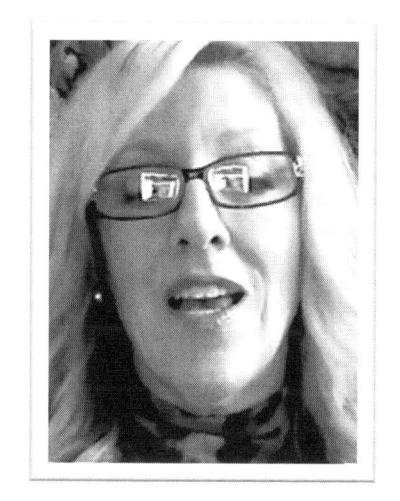

It was tolerable until one morning four years ago when I was jogging on a treadmill, as I did every morning. I was on incline when suddenly I was not able to breathe. I ended up in an emergency room.

In hospital I was given lots of medication (steroids as well as other types of asthma medicine), but it did not work; in fact, it made me feel worse.

When I returned home, I was not able to get out of bed; if I tried, I was out of breath. If I ate too much or sometimes if I simply ate, I was not able to breathe. My breathlessness was almost constant as well as my fatigue. I kept visiting doctors who did all kinds of tests. First, the assumption was that the cause of my breathing trouble was my heart, but it was proven that it was not. In fact, every test came back normal. I did not know what to do! After a while, I became able to leave the bed and move on to a couch. Nevertheless, it was a time when all I was able to do is sitting on a couch.

I started searching the Internet and found a holistic doctor who told me that the problem was my thyroid. He prescribed me several types of medication (including steroids) and recommended vitamins and supplements. Nothing worked! A year and a half passed and I was feeling worse, but the doctor kept convincing me that I should stay on this medication longer and eventually it would help. I believed him, but it did not work. Eventually, two years later I started tapering myself off this medication.

Meanwhile, I kept searching the Internet and finally found on Amazon, Sasha's DVD-set *The Breathing Normalization Method*. I ordered it and watched all five discs. In the first one, Sasha was sharing a story of Thomas, her husband, whose asthma was severe. Listening to his story, I thought, "Oh, my goodness, there is someone like me out there, and he was able to overcome his predicament."

Step-by-step I started implementing all instructions in the DVD. After three months of doing this, my health significantly improved. I was doing fairly well when all of a sudden I had a setback, and at this time I decided to contact the Breathing Center.

Eventually, I started working one-on-one with Sasha via Skype. Breathing Normalization changed my life! I was not only able to get off the couch but get on a treadmill. I thought there was no way for me to be on a treadmill ever again… and yet during my Breathing Normalization training, following Sasha's instructions, I would start every day on my treadmill. First, it was a bit hard to control my breathing while walking, but I learned how to do it. As a result, I became much healthier and stronger. And I kept feeling better and getting stronger every day!

Breathing Normalization was the only thing I found which helped me to overcome my asthma. Since I was young, I had seen so many doctors, but no one ever mentioned that I could overcome my breathing problems so simply. So thank you to Doctor Buteyko who developed this approach, and Sasha and Thomas, who made it available in the States. It saved my life! Now, I am able to lead a normal life!

22. Breathing Center's Student
Denver, CO

Part 1, written in 2010:
I'm 13 years old and I've had bad asthma all of my life. I went to all types of doctors for years on end, while taking various medications that didn't seem to be doing anything. About a month ago, my parents discovered an article in *The New York Times* about Buteyko Center USA (Breathing Center), so we decided to try it out.

When I first started Breathing Normalization, my body was in bad condition. My nose was always badly stuffed up, and I would breathe heavily out of my mouth all the time. If I ran up a big hill, or just went for a jog, I would need my inhaler. My body could handle exercise, but it could not handle my asthma.

When I arrived at the Center, I could barely do a breath hold of 3 seconds! Now, a month later, I can easily do a breath hold of 20 seconds. And my nose is clear most of the time, for the first time in my life! Each week I got on my computer and worked online with one of the practitioners and did my exercises with his instructions. By changing my diet and practicing the exercises, I have greatly improved in a very short period of time. And now I can run three miles without difficulty! Thanks to the Center!

Part 2, written in 2016:
I am 19 years old now and have not been suffering from asthma since I took Breathing Normalization training in the Center. My doctor told me that I don't have asthma anymore because I outgrew it.

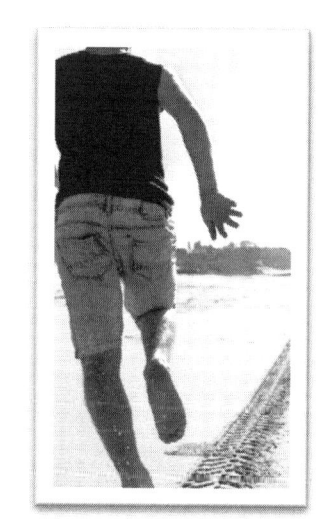

23. Gurusahay Khalsa
Dunwoody, GA, 2010

Dear Thomas,

I wanted to thank you for sharing the Buteyko Method with me. It's one of the most amazing things I have ever done in my life. I learned of the Buteyko Method many years ago and even bought a tape from Australia on how to do the method. For some reason, I never watched it in its entirety and never applied the techniques even though I suffered from asthma.

As I explained when we first talked, I have had asthma and have used an inhaler at least twice a day for nearly 30 years, essentially all my adult life.

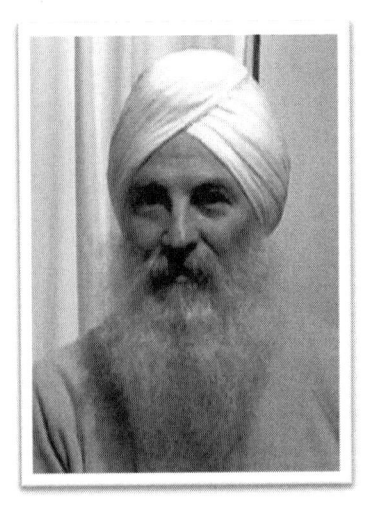

I am a holistic chiropractor, an acupuncturist and nutritionist in private practice since 1978. I have been a Kundalini Yoga practitioner and teacher for over 35 years and, as you know, breathing techniques are an integral part of yoga. I have studied these wonderful healing arts out of a passion for understanding the road to health to help my patients, and I have diligently applied what I've learned to help heal myself. I have attempted to correct my asthma all these years with all these techniques, with no permanent relief.

A few months ago a friend sent me the *New York Times* article on Buteyko Center USA. I saw the title, Buteyko, and filed it away for future reading. After all, near the very top of my goal list for the last 30 years I wrote, "study and implement Buteyko" but never took the necessary actions steps.

While I was studying to teach yogic breathing techniques to future yoga teachers in November of 2009, I ran across a statement from my yoga teacher to practice a specific mantra that "would solve all breathing problems." I committed to chanting the mantra daily for 31 minutes and sat back waiting for the results.

Four or five days later I stumbled upon the *New York Times* article buried in my inbox and decided to call your center "right now" to find a local referral for a practitioner to finally start learning and implementing the Buteyko Method. To my dismay, you said there was no local teacher but that we could do long distance learning via the internet. I reluctantly agreed to give it a shot, my hopes and prayers for resolution of my asthma and my newly found mantra prodding me on.

During the fall of 2009, my asthma had taken a turn for the worse, prompting me to use my rescue inhaler three or four times a week in addition to my preventative inhaler. I even went to a new doctor to see about getting a different prescription, dreading the idea of having to take an inhaler with steroids.

Within a few days of our first session, I stopped needing my rescue inhaler but continued on with my Buteyko practices, encouraged. After a few weeks I felt stabilized, but I still needed the preventative inhaler twice a day and started feeling discouraged. After all, maybe this Buteyko Method wasn't good enough to cure my asthma completely in six weeks, even though I'd suffered nearly 30 years! Strange how impatience makes us think funny things.

During our next consultation I expressed my frustration, and you patiently explained that the Buteyko practices had to actually be done three times a day (as you had instructed me) and that I should have patience. Within a few days of re-committing to my exercises, my asthma dramatically improved, and my need for the inhalers dramatically decreased. With my doctor's blessing, I was able to completely wean myself from the inhalers.

It's been over six weeks now since I've last used an inhaler. I still do my breathing and relaxation exercises three times a day, and I still stick to my diet fastidiously. And I've clearly recognized that when my chest feels tight, when I feel like I might have an attack, I can just take a break, do my breathing and the attack will stop. Even though the chiropractic, acupuncture and dietary/supplement regimens I received all helped some, the breathing was the key component to my relief.

This is a miracle. I thank you and your staff from the depths of my being. I only pray that all people who suffer from any kind of breathing difficulties find this wonderful method and can be relieved from the burden of inhaling their life from a drug instead of breathing easily, freely and consciously through their own healed bodies.

24. Paul Hixson
Urbana, Illinois, 2016

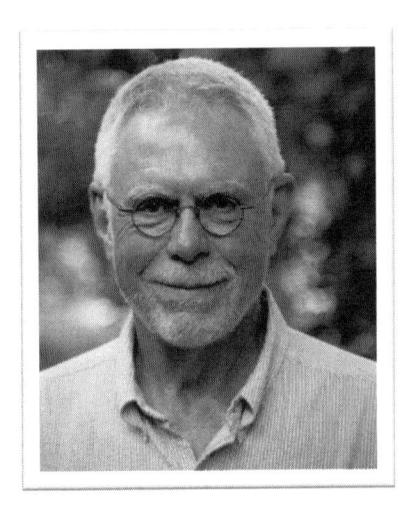

I am a 70-year-old man, and I'm happy to report that due to learning and applying the principles of the Buteyko Breathing Normalization method, as taught to me by the great staff of the Breathing Center, I am currently enjoying excellent health. But that definitely was not always the case.

In fact, I had lived with significant breathing problems pretty much my whole life, up until about two years ago. As a child, I had lots of allergy related "summer colds" that seemed to always end in endless coughing bouts and a burning feeling in my chest. I was never able to run as far or fast as other kids my age, and when I tried, I would end up gasping for breath. I seemed to catch more colds that most of my classmates, and they definitely lasted longer. In hindsight, I now realize that I breathed through my mouth a lot, but I had no idea at the time that that was bad for me.

As a young adult, the pattern morphed into one in which I averaged about 5-6 colds a year, and most of them ended in prolonged periods of uncontrollable coughing that would often last weeks after the main cold had subsided. In my late 20s and early 30s my family physician began pulling me out of those prolonged coughing attacks by using an injectable steroid called Depo-Medrol. At first those shots were amazingly successful, but soon they seemed to lose much of their effectiveness.

When I was 38, I experienced a terrible respiratory crisis as a result of working around a land reclamation project where dozens of large bulldozers and trenching machines were digging up the earth. I went into absolutely unstoppable coughing attacks that left me totally incapacitated for a number of days. The Depo-Medrol shots didn't work—nothing worked. I ended up in the hospital for two weeks on IV's and spent the following three weeks at home recovering.

After switching to the care of a lung specialist, I was told that, "you have asthma", and for the next 30 years I was treated as an asthmatic. Over the following three decades, I ended up taking nearly every type of drug that conventional western medicine offers to combat asthma—bronchodilators, inhaled nasal steroids, inhaled steroids for the lungs, plus rescue inhalers. Nonetheless, my health pattern still remained that of catching several colds a year, with most of them going into full-blown coughing asthma at the end of the cold. And then most of those colds had to be followed by a tapered course of Prednisone tablets (often accompanied by the Depo-Medrol injections). Despite leading an otherwise active life, that was pretty much the norm for the next thirty years.

Then, in November 2014, shortly after retiring from a long career at a major Midwestern university, I came down with a cold that went into the worst asthma attack I had ever experienced. At the time of that attack, I had been taking the following medicines on a daily basis: Theophylline, Nasacort, Symbicort, Singulair, and Albuterol. And when the cold turned into asthma, I was additionally put on a 40 mg taper-down dosage of Prednisone and also given a Depo-Medrol injection. But nothing helped. I couldn't even sleep because if I lay down in bed, I would quickly begin an uncontrollable coughing bout that would last for several hours.

In desperation, I turned to the web, hoping to find some new "miracle drug" for dealing with asthma. Fortunately, instead I came across the article by *New York Times* health columnist, Jane Brody, referred to earlier in this book, which, in turn, led me to the website of the Breathing Center. That turned out to be a blessing. After downloading the Buteyko Breathing Manual and reading for the first time, that the true cause of my asthma was continual over-breathing (initially, a very counter-intuitive idea), I next realized that although I could grasp the theory of why I needed to breathe less, I still needed the guidance of a personal trainer to teach me how to actually do this.

I ended up taking both the Level One and Level Two online courses with Robert Operman and Sasha Yakovleva respectively. Both were excellent instructors, and now, more than a year later, I can truly say that learning Breathing Normalization has given me my health back. In fact, *my health is now better than it has ever been*. By the time I had finished the Level One course, I was already off of all the maintenance asthma meds that I had been taking for 30 years. In that Level One course, I learned how to change my 68-year habit of mouth breathing (including while talking and while sleeping); I learned to change my diet; and I resumed a rigorous exercise program. During that 8-week Level One course, I went from a nearly non-existent control pause of 2 seconds to around 20 seconds. By the end of my Level Two course, I had addressed several other underlying causes of what Dr. Buteyko called "chroniosepsis" and, as a result, my control pause had increased to 30+ seconds. I was a new man.

In the year since my online trainings, I have continued to apply the teachings of the Breathing Center on a daily basis. I have accelerated my physical activities and now walk an average of a little under 8 miles every day (something I could never have done before). Based on the readings of my personal tracking device, in the last 19 weeks, I've actually logged a little over 1,000 miles just walking around my hometown. I have not taken any asthma meds in 16 months; nor have I had any asthma problems. I sleep more soundly and rest more fully than ever before. I've only had one cold in the past year and it was just a regular 7-day cold -- the sort that a normal "healthy person" has with no asthma at the tail end. My seasonal inhalant allergies are significantly less bothersome, and my blood pressure is much better than it has been for years. It's remarkable; but at this point I am truly asthma free and in the best over-all health of my life. I owe that all to the breakthrough discoveries of Dr. Buteyko, the encouragement of my family physician, and the wonderful teaching staff at the Breathing Center.

Part 2: Questions And Answers About Asthma

Below you will see questions asthmatics and their relatives often ask at the Breathing Center in the United States and the Clinica Buteyko in Moscow, Russia.

Q: How to pronounce the word "Buteyko"?

A: Many people pronounce this word as "bu'teyko"- similar to the word "beauty". This pronunciation is incorrect! It should be pronounced as "boo - teyko"- similar to the word "boot."

Q: Do I over-breathe? How can I check to see if I hyperventilate or not?

A: The best way to check if you hyperventilate is to visit the Breathing Test page at www.breathingcenter.com. There, you can learn how to measure your Control Pause and Positive Maximum Pause and submit the results of your test for review. You will receive a free evaluation report based on your results.

Q: People with breathing difficulties are often told to take a deep breath. Is this wrong?

A: Yes. While the concept of deep breathing, or 'just take a deep breath,' has become a part of the popular Western culture, excessive breathing is harmful, especially for people with breathing difficulties. Dr. Buteyko pointed out (based on the Bohr Effect) that oxygenation of the vital organs reduces as breathing increases. In fact, over-breathing can provoke an asthma attack or other breathing problems.

Q: Will I suffocate if I breathe less?

A: No, if you know how to do it. For most students who are new to Buteyko Breathing Normalization, the concept of breathing reduction may seem counter-intuitive. Many have spent their lives fighting to breathe enough air. However, breathing less triggers a relaxation and dilation of the smooth muscles along the bronchial tubes, which gives an asthmatic relief from their symptoms.

Q: I've read about Dr. Buteyko's breathing method. Is it a good idea to start experimenting with breathing reduction on my own?

A: Dr. Buteyko always insisted that his method was best learned under the supervision of a competent practitioner. Attempting to retrain your breathing on your own could be hazardous to your health, or you may not have strong positive results. It is always better to seek expert supervision at Breathing Center in the US or Clinica Buteyko in Moscow.

Having said that, we also need to mention that the Breathing Center's website offers various educational materials—DVDs, CDs and books. While they do not replace the need for being trained by a Breathing Normalization Specialist, they offer an opportunity to learn the method on your own in a safe and effective way if you follow the instructions precisely.

Q: Which of Breathing Center's programs are best for asthmatics?

A: The most effective program is called Full Training, which is a part of our Level 1 Breathing Normalization courses. This program is available online and can be taken by adults or children from anywhere in the world. Full Training is a so-called "all-inclusive program" because everything you need to improve your breathing and overall health is included in this course. The main part of the package contains weekly sessions with a Breathing Normalization Specialist who tailors the method to your individual needs and gives you unlimited support after completion of this program.

Q: Can Breathing Normalization help with various breathing difficulties?

A: Absolutely! Dr. Buteyko's discovery and breathing method both revolve around balancing the body's use of oxygen and carbon dioxide. It is the imbalance of these two elements that causes the reactions of the body, which, in turn, create the majority of breathing difficulties people experience. By applying Buteyko Breathing Normalization properly, the system balance is restored and breathing difficulties defeated.

Q: What are Dr. Buteyko's breathing exercises?

A: The breathing exercises are the core element of the Buteyko Breathing Normalization Method, which is a natural, drug-free, holistic technique to help people suffering from asthma, allergies and breathing difficulties, as well as many other health issues. The exercises were developed by Dr. Konstantin Buteyko, as well as his wife, Ludmila Buteyko, and her son, Andrey Novozhilov, MD. Some of the exercises were further advanced at the Breathing Center in the US. Many clinical trials have shown that Dr. Buteyko's breathing exercises can safely reduce asthma symptoms such as coughing, wheezing, excessive mucus, suffocation attacks and the need for reliever medication; they also greatly increase the overall quality of life. Breathing exercises are most successful when tailored to the client's individual condition and rate of improvement.

Q: Can you give me any advice right now?

A: Yes. Always breathe gently and through your nose only. This will greatly reduce hyperventilation, which, as Dr. Buteyko discovered, is the major contributing factor into the development of asthma, breathing difficulties and lung problems.

Q: I wake up each morning with a stuffy nose; will this method help me?

A: Yes, if you apply it! By making your nose stuffy, your body protects itself from over-breathing; it simply narrows airways. You need to learn how to reduce your breathing, and that will eliminate the root of your problem. Aside from that, it is useful to learn and apply a special technique, which Dr. Buteyko developed for clearing nasal passages. You can use it any time you feel a need to unblock your nose. It is a gentle technique and, unlike many others, does not cause additional hyperventilation and mucus creation.

Q: Will asthma continue to appear in my family if I use Dr. Buteyko's approach?

A: According to Dr. Buteyko, asthma as a disease cannot be passed from parents to children. However, given a tendency to bronchospasm, the body's defense mechanism against an excessive loss of CO2 can be inherited. In families of asthmatics there are often children without asthma symptoms who have developed different defense mechanisms—for example, the ability of the blood vessels to spasm. This can lead to high blood pressure in later life. At the Clinica Buteyko Moscow and the Breathing Center, practitioners have helped many people to stop asthma being passed from generation to generation.

Q: I have had asthma for 40 years. I am on inhaled steroids and rescue inhalers. Can Buteyko Breathing Normalization help me?

A: Many of clients in the Clinica Buteyko Moscow and the Breathing Center have had asthma since childhood. According to Dr. Buteyko, the root cause of asthma is hyperventilation. Once a student has eliminated his hyperventilation—no matter how long he has had asthma—he or she will lose most or all of his symptoms. Many students become completely drug-free.

Q: My daughter has asthma. I am worried about the long-term effects of medication and about her suffering from asthma her whole life. Can Breathing Normalization help?

A: Definitely. The Breathing Normalization method can be successfully taught to children of all ages. In fact, children often understand the method much more quickly than adults, and can shift their breathing and asthma symptoms more easily than adults can. However, in most cases, a parent or guardian must learn the method alongside their child, in order to support and mentor their child outside of the formal sessions.

Q: My son has asthma. My other son has allergies and my husband snores. I think we could all benefit from learning Breathing Normalization. Can families attend educational programs together?

A: Yes. At the Breathing Center, all immediate family members may attend programs together. While attention will be paid primarily to the asthmatic student (child) for whom the family enrolled, all family members will have the opportunity to learn the method and improve their health. We highly encourage families to take educational courses together, as this creates the best environment for the primary student (child), and all other family members, to benefit from this method.

Q: I am planning on having a baby. My first child is asthmatic, and I don't want the next one to suffer from breathing difficulties. Can Breathing Normalization help?

A: We strongly recommend all women who are planning on becoming pregnant to learn how to normalize their breathing. It is much easier to give birth to a healthy baby than it is to improve the health of a baby who is born unhealthy. Applying Breathing Normalization before pregnancy will ensure that your child will not be born as a hyperventilator. According to Dr. Buteyko, if a child is born with good breathing, then he or she is in perfect health.

Q: What is the core principal of the Dr. Buteyko's approach?

A: Dr. Konstantin Pavlovich Buteyko, a renowned Soviet scientist working in Russia, created a revolutionary theory that asthma symptoms (as well as many other types of breathing problems) are the result of chronic hyperventilation. Physiologically, asthma is characterized by both chronic inflammation in the lungs and bronchial spasm. Severe asthma and COPD are further characterized by structural damage to the lungs, leading to poor gas exchange in the alveoli (air sacs). Dr. Buteyko's theory was that the deep/heavy breathing of asthmatics (chronic hyperventilation or over-breathing) and the coughing, wheezing, chest pain, mucus and suffocation attacks (asthmatic symptoms) are related in a unique way.

Based on the laws of physiology, we know that hyperventilation depletes the level of CO_2 in the lungs. While CO_2 is a by-product of metabolism, and some needs to be removed from the body, it is in fact an absolutely essential component of life, which regulates many functions in the human body. To begin with, proper oxygenation of the brain, heart, kidneys and other vital organs and tissues relies on appropriate amounts of CO2 remaining in the body (due to the Bohr Effect). When CO2 levels fall below a certain threshold, the body experiences systemic oxygen deprivation. This is very dangerous for the body. Dr. Buteyko theorized that acute and chronically low CO2 levels in the lungs can cause pH shifts in the body, which create a cascade of negative biochemical reactions, with deleterious effects on metabolism, the immune and nervous systems, and most other body systems.

Dr. Buteyko's theory is that chronic hyperventilation is so dangerous and damaging to human health that the body creates defensive/survival mechanisms in order to adapt to this constant stress. Asthmatic symptoms (coughing, wheezing, chest pain, excessive mucus and suffocation attacks) may in fact be a defensive/survival mechanism to protect against over-breathing. Specifically, these symptoms, unpleasant and scary as they may be, have an overall effect of reducing respiration, and therefore maintain alveolar CO2 levels within an acceptable range. Though these symptoms can cause great suffering, this mechanism actually allows the body to maintain essential biological constants necessary to life.

Dr. Buteyko thought that modern pharmaceutical treatments to eliminate bronchial spasm, though effective in temporarily removing symptoms, were, in fact, disturbing the body's defensive/survival mechanism. This may explain why asthma symptoms often get worse with prolonged medicating. Over time, medication may be creating an even more powerful asthmatic response in order to maintain the body's protective mechanism. However, Dr. Buteyko theorized, if hyperventilation could be eliminated, and breathing normalized, then perhaps the symptoms of asthma and other breathing difficulties would no longer be 'needed' by the body to protect itself.

This is the central principle of Dr. Buteyko's approach for the treatment of asthma and other breathing difficulties. By systematically normalizing air consumption and consequently CO2 levels in the lungs, through the use of the Buteyko breathing exercises and certain lifestyle changes, Dr. Buteyko found that symptoms of asthma could be tamed, a profound healing could take place in the lungs, and a person could regain their health.

Q: Is yawning a source of hyperventilation?

A: Contrary to a common assumption, Dr. Buteyko considered yawning being an exception from a harmful effect of mouth breathing and hyperventilation. Yawning helps to normalize gas exchange and often follows relaxation. Many people who start practicing Buteyko Breathing Normalization, experience intense yawning, which is considered being a sign that the method is applied effectively. To control this reaction is a mistake. The advice to "yawn with your mouth closed" contradicts Dr. Buteyko's work.

Q: What is the worst physical activity for an asthmatic?

A: For many asthmatics, the most dangerous physical activity is swimming, since in most cases it is accompanied by mouth breathing and excessive breathing. This could lead to a significant loss of CO_2 and trigger asthma symptoms. Nevertheless, if a person "breathes less" during swimming, this activity could become very beneficial.

Q: What is the best type of physical activities for asthmatics?

A: On the initial stages of Breathing Normalization training, it is walking and eventually running. Any physical activity should be performed by breathing gently or relatively gently through the nose only.

Q: According to this method, "deep breathing" is bad for health and "shallow breathing" is good. Is this correct?

A: Breathing Normalization Specialists always try to avoid usage of these terms since they could be rather confusing. It is true that excessive breathing is harmful when gentle, invisible breathing is healthful. The terms "deep" and "shallow" breathing are often used in conjunction with the Buteyko Method as literal (but not correct) translation from Russian of the terms used by Dr. Buteyko in his work. The Buteyko Method is concerned with an overall consumption of air and increase of the CO2 level in the lungs. Sometimes this result could be achieved by slow and therefore long inhalation and exhalation (which is sometimes called "deep breathing") but cannot be achieved by rapid chest breathing, which is often evident in case of asthma and COPD (sometimes it is called "shallow breathing).

Q: Do I need to practice reduced breathing day and night?

A: You should try your best to correct your breathing every time you notice that you are breathing excessively. Breathing Normalization Specialists train people to control their breathing 24 hours. As a result of this training, eventually people are able to maintain reduced breathing automatically throughout day and night.

Q: Should I stop playing soccer and other sports until my breathing is healed and my asthma is gone?

A: If you are not able to breathe through your nose while being physically active, you should stop playing this sport until your breathing is improved. When you are able to do this physical activity while breathing through your nose, you can come back to it. In this case instead of being harmful for your health, it will become beneficial. This is especially important in case of children.

Q: What is the worst type of food for breathing?

A: In most cases dairy products and various forms of meat trigger hyperventilation.

Q: Is eating chocolate bad for my asthma?

A: Not necessarily. Some people have strong individual reactions to chocolate, and in this case it can trigger asthma symptoms. Most asthmatics don't have this reaction. Observe your breathing after eating chocolate or any other sugary products and decide for yourself.

Q: What beverages are helpful for asthma?

A: Dr. Buteyko recommended drinking plenty of pure water and nothing else.

Q: I have heard that it is beneficial to eat salt if a person hyperventilates. Is it true?

A: Yes. Salt, especially Himalayan rock salt, is an important part of the Breathing Normalization process.

Q: My son started practicing *Steps* following recommendations of one of the Buteyko books he found on Amazon. He thought that this exercise would stop his asthma, but it made it worse. What went wrong?

A: That is why it is important to apply this method under supervision of a Breathing Normalization Specialist. Unfortunately, this situation is rather common. People who learn *Steps Exercise* from some books often end up with negative results because they practice breath holds too intensely, which triggers hyperventilation.

Q: I am not capable of setting up time for formal breathing exercises. Does it mean that Breathing Normalization is not for me?

A: No. You can practice Buteyko Breathing Normalization informally by incorporating it into any of your daily activities. Usually, a Breathing Normalization Specialist discusses with a client his or her daily routine and helps to turn it into a chain of breathing exercises. Generally speaking, doing a lot of short breath holds throughout the day is very beneficial. Also, try to start each day with a walk or any other physical activities combined with nasal breathing and preferably breathing exercises. For as long as your Control Pause is increasing, you are improving your breathing.

Q: In yoga classes, students are often instructed to force their breath. Is it good for asthmatics?

A: The approach towards breathing in traditional hatha yoga in India is very different compared to its American version. Traditionally, yoga students were advised to breathe gently and through the nose only, which is in harmony with Dr. Buteyko's method. Pranayama of yoga of breathing was taught only to healthy and strong people whose CP (by our hypothesis) was much higher than average.

In a modern Western yoga class, the recommendations to take a deep breath, force your breathing, to breathe non-stop and breathe through the mouth, often lead to worsening of asthma and allergies and can trigger the development of various breathing difficulties. The traditional yoga is supportive of breathing reduction, increase of CO_2 and health improvement.

Q: What affect can my spiritual practice have on my asthma?

A: The correlation between a spiritual practice and breathing is not a part of this book; however, it was an important part of Dr. Buteyko's work, and it is one of the key elements in Breathing Normalization training. Generally speaking, authentic prayers, chanting, and bowing combined with nasal breathing increase the CO_2 level significantly.

Q: Will I experience oxygen starvation if I attempt to breathe less?

A: Quiet opposite. By reducing air consumption, oxygenation of the whole body increases. As a result, a person experiences more energy, more mental clarity and focus, and less physical discomfort.

Q: More air I take in, more oxygen my body receives, correct?

A: No. Learn about the Bohr effect to realize that it works the other way around. Less air we take in, more oxygen gets released by hemoglobin to all cells. No matter how much oxygen we inhale, we are not going to receive a sufficient amount unless the level of CO_2 in the lungs is normal. The level of CO_2 regulates how much oxygen is released.

Q: In various books, I have read different instructions on measuring the Control Pause. I am confused over whether to measure the CP after inhaling, after exhaling, or as some authors describe, with the diaphragm in a relatively neutral position—so neither breathing overly in or out. Which one is right?

A: You measure the Control Pause or Positive Maximum Pause when you are fully relaxed after a normal exhalation. When you are completely relaxed, you automatically pause your breathing for a moment after exhaling. This is the exact point from which to measure the CP. However, it is very common for many people to have difficulty in sensing this point because they fail to relax sufficiently. They tend to force the out breath and inhale a little extra before they measure the CP. Although the CP measured in this way will not be accurate, this is not something to get too concerned about. Do your best to relax and to start to hold your breath at the unforced end of a normal exhalation and resume breathing at the first urge to breathe. Concentrate on measuring your CP consistently so that every time you take a measure it is done in exactly the same way. This will ensure that the trend of your readings provides correct feedback on your progress. Even if you are not measuring your CP absolutely correctly, as long as it is increasing you will know you are on the right track. The more you measure your CP and practice the exercises the more skillful you will become at feeling your breathing, and the more accurate your CP measurement will become.

Q: There are many excellent athletes who eat healthily and are physically very active but still have asthma. Why is that?

A: The reason is that while athletes may achieve a high level of fitness and exercise strenuously, they tend to force the out breath or inhale excessively. The CO_2 produced by their muscles is less than the amount ventilated. This imbalance can arise whether they are exercising strongly or not and can trigger asthma symptoms as a defense mechanism. When exercising, the muscles will generate large quantities of CO_2. However, this will be more than matched by an increase in breathing. They should, therefore, do Buteyko breathing exercises to establish a balance between CO_2 production and their breathing.

Q: It seems to me that there is a major contradiction in Dr. Buteyko's approach. Exercise # 1 aims to reduce breathing through relaxation, but other exercises involve conscious control to reduce breathing by generating a feeling of air shortage, which results in tension. How can the two be reconciled?

A: There is no contradiction in the objective to reduce breathing. Both approaches will achieve this aim, but by different ways, which over time should converge. It is preferable to reduce breathing through relaxation, as this is a more pleasant experience than doing breath-holds. However, the Buteyko Method™ recognizes that many people find it difficult to reduce breathing through relaxation alone, especially if they have a low CP, and consequently, low CO2. Low CO2 causes the nervous system to become overly sensitized, leading to feelings of tension, anxiety and nervousness. This can make it extremely difficult to relax. The Buteyko Method™, therefore, incorporates other exercises involving conscious control and that do not depend primarily on relaxation. Students who initially follow the conscious control route usually progressively learn how to follow the relaxation method once their CP starts to improve significantly.

Q: Is it really possible to reduce breathing through relaxation? Do you have any evidence to prove this?

A: It is well known that relaxation techniques such as meditation can profoundly affect physiological processes.

Various studies have shown that meditation induces a host of biochemical and physical changes in the body, collectively referred to as the "relaxation response." The relaxation response includes changes in metabolism, lowering of heart rate, respiration, blood pressure and changes in brain chemistry.

Meditation, as in Exercise # 1, normally involves avoiding wandering thoughts and fantasies, and calming and focusing the mind. This state of relaxation is qualitatively of a different order than the common understanding of relaxation, like sitting in front of the TV watching a movie and eating a pizza. This will not result in the physiological change that accompanies profound relaxation achievable through meditation and Exercise # 1.

Exercise # 1 is really another version of meditation using the focus on breathing and relaxation of the breathing muscles as the means for avoiding wandering thoughts. Some teachers of meditation and relaxation techniques suggest that the breathing pattern should be changed, including taking deep breaths. This should of course be avoided. It is sufficient to relax deeply to induce an automatic reduction in breathing.

Q: What is the physiological basis of relaxation and stress?

A: The body is governed by the nervous system. The body has two basic states: one of activity and energy to overcome threats and fight to survive, which is governed by the sympathetic nervous system; the other of recuperation and relaxation, governed by the parasympathetic system. Both systems are actually operational all the time, but with one or the other tending to dominate.

The sympathetic system is responsible for the provision of energy needed especially in situations like hunger, fear, or extreme physical activity. After having mastered such a challenging situation, the body is exhausted and needs to rest, recover and gain new energy. These tasks are under the control of the parasympathetic system. Basically, the parasympathetic nerves influence organs to restore and to save energy. Exercise # 1, as with other relaxation techniques, induces an increase in the parasympathetic tone.

Q: I have read in an academic study about the effectiveness of the Buteyko Method that members of the control group who only concerned themselves with relaxation did not reach any significant improvement in their state of health, while the group that applied the Buteyko Method, achieved a great improvement in health. Should I conclude that relaxation alone is ineffective in improving asthma?

A: There definitely was some improvement in the control group. For example, there was a reduction in their use of bronchodilators. But the changes were insignificant compared to the reduction achieved in the Buteyko group. In the control group, the patients were not told to keep their breathing to a minimum. Without this information, relaxation alone was much less effective. As mentioned above, it is also likely that the relaxation group found it difficult to fully relax if they already had a relatively low CP. If the CP is low, it is often difficult to relax sufficiently because of the excited state of the nervous system caused by low CO2.

Q: Dr. Novozhilov warns that it is difficult to learn Buteyko just by reading the book and following the instructions and that it is desirable to learn the method from a Breathing Normalization Specialist. Yet the book nevertheless describes in detail how the exercises should be performed. Is it safe for me to try to do the exercises without the supervision of a practitioner?

A: It is preferable to learn the method from a Breathing Normalization Specialist. In the USA, you can find a practitioner through the Breathing Center, which officially represents the Clinica Buteyko in Moscow. The staff will connect a student with the right practitioner. Although it is not always possible to find someone who teaches the method nearby, the Breathing Center offers courses online, via Skype, so a student can learn from anywhere in the world. Andrey Novozhilov is one of the online consultants.

This manual serves as an introduction and prevents students from making basic mistakes. Patients should always stay in touch with their family doctor and make sure that he or she is following up with them and keeping track of changes made to their medication, so as to avoid any possible health risks.

If you are unsupervised, you are strongly advised to stick to the exercises described in this book. If your health deteriorates or if your breathing seems to destabilize and becomes chaotic, you should immediately stop the exercises and seek the guidance of a Breathing Normalization Specialist.

The Buteyko approach seems deceptively easy to learn, but there are many subtleties and complexities that can arise and are best dealt with by an experienced practitioner. Learning the Buteyko Method is somewhat similar to learning yoga. Like all these disciplines, it is dependent on the "apprentice" learning from an expert in the craft. It is possible to learn the basics by reading a book, but it is extremely rare to become a master of any of these disciplines, including Buteyko, without, at some stage, having somebody already proficient in the art show you how to do it. An expert, outside observer is much better placed to identify and correct the many mistakes that are easily made—sometimes big, often small, and sometimes having to do with lifestyle as much as how an exercise is performed.

Q: How to find and choose a Buteyko teacher?

A: In order to find a certified Breathing Normalization Specialist who teaches the Buteyko method online or in your area, visit www.breathingcenter.com and check the list of Breathing Normalization Specialists worldwide. Practitioners listed on this site have the proper education and legal rights to teach the Buteyko breathing method. If you have found a practitioner through another source, please be very careful. Unfortunately, anyone can call himself a certified Buteyko Practitioner, but this does not mean that a person received the proper training, or was accredited by Clinica Buteyko Moscow to teach the method. We sincerely hope that it the future this situation will improve.

Q: I don't know how I can make use of the recommendations regarding the steroid protocol. They seem to be written for Russian conditions only. In my country, asthmatics usually do not take steroids in tablet form. Instead they are given a prescription for a steroid inhaler to be used twice a day, giving always the same dose. It is impossible to break my dose into thirds. How do I use such an inhaler to adjust my dose in the manner described by the author?

A: That is exactly one of the problems with the steroid inhalers and the reason why Dr. Novozhilov recommends taking steroids in tablet form. With inhalers, it is not possible to set the 24-hour dose accurately and then regulate the dose into fractions of your 24-hour dose. You could try to adapt the use of the inhaler, for example by using it once in the morning and twice at night, but this would be a crude method, less likely to set the correct 24-hour dose and the subsequent dosing regimen than if you were using oral steroids. You should consult your doctor about this question and ask him to choose the right medicine for you.

Q: I have been using an inhaler that gives me a combination of cortisone and a bronchodilator in one dose. There is no way for me to keep these two active substances apart. This means that I am unable to tell how many puffs of a bronchodilator I need per day. The bronchodilator, which is incorporated in my inhaler, lasts for 12 hours. What should I do?

A: Dr. Novozhilov recommends to talk to your doctor and ask for separate bronchodilator and steroid puffers rather than accept these combination packs. You should probably change to one of the "old" applications, where you take your bronchodilator and steroids separately. These new applicators, which combine both substances, as practical as they may seem, only help to complicate matters. See your doctor about this, and tell him about Dr. Buteyko's approach.

Q: How is a Breathing Normalization Specialist is going to treat my asthma?

A: At Clinica Buteyko Moscow, the Buteyko Method is taught by medical doctors. In the US, Buteyko teachers certified by Clinica Buteyko Moscow are called Breathing Normalization Specialists; they are trained by Dr. Novozhilov and other Russian Buteyko-doctors; however, Breathing Normalization Specialists are not medical professionals and therefore do not treat any particular disease.

Breathing Normalization Specialists educate people on Dr. Buteyko's breathing method and teach them how to reduce or eliminate over-breathing. Ordinarily, Breathing Normalization leads to significant improvement in many bodily systems and their overall functioning. As a result, a person becomes much healthier and commonly loses their primary symptoms. In case of asthmatics, asthma symptoms often become reduced or stopped completely.

Q: Will Breathing Normalization specialists advise on when to stop taking my medicine?

A: At the Clinica Buteyko Moscow, doctors will do that. In the US, the Breathing Normalization Specialists are not medical doctors and do not give advice regarding medication. They help their students to normalize their breathing, and as a result, students often lose most or all asthma symptoms. Decisions about medication and dosing are between students and their primary health physician. However, often when symptoms are reduced, and standard medical diagnostics deems the asthmatic condition improving, physicians will recommend a reduction in medication.

Q: I have coughing fits, wheezing, suffocation attacks, excessive mucus, etc. Can the Buteyko Breathing Normalization help with these symptoms?

A: Yes. Dr. Buteyko discovered that chronic hyperventilation could be very dangerous or even lethal. In order to protect itself, the body creates various defense mechanisms to reduce hyperventilation. Coughing, wheezing, suffocation attacks, excessive mucus, and stuffy nose are just a few of these mechanisms. The purpose of each of these "symptoms" is to reduce hyperventilation, thereby protecting the body from even greater harm. When a person reduces his or her hyperventilation voluntarily, the body no longer relies on these symptoms as a means to prevent hyperventilation. Many people greatly reduce symptoms within the first few weeks of taking breathing re-training; after completing the program, many people lose their symptoms completely.

Q: I have a lot of questions about the Breathing Normalization Method, but I want to speak to a real person. How can I do this?

A: We encourage any and all questions you have about Dr. Buteyko's work and our educational programs. The best forum for your questions is our free Preliminary Consultation available to anyone who is considering taking our Breathing Normalization training. This is a one-hour conversation with a Breathing Normalization Specialist by telephone, Skype or in person, during which you can discuss your situation and the possible application of the method in detail.

Part 3: Breathing Normalization Products And Services

These products are available at the online store at BreathingCenter.com

DVD and Downloads

The Breathing Normalization Method. Learn Buteyko To Stop Breathing Difficulties and Improve Health

Session # 1: Breathing Awareness: Mouth Vs. Nose Breathing

This video is the first session of the 5-disc video training, which is a complete step-by-step self-help program on the Buteyko Breathing Normalization Method suitable for adults and children. Watching this video session, you will learn about Dr. Buteyko's approach, how to evaluate your breathing in order to evaluate your health, the healing crisis, nasal breathing versus mouth breathing, and more. All sessions contain demonstrations of breathing exercises and recommendations on when and how to do them.

Session # 2: Hidden Sources of Hyperventilation - Breathing During Sleep, Stress And While Talking

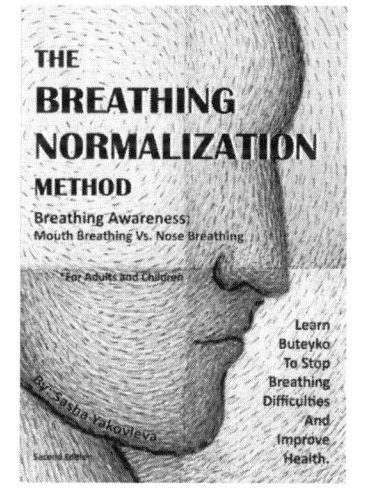

Session # 3: Food, Water And Beverages - Choose A Diet Conducive To Reduced Breathing

Session # 4: Breathing And Physical Exercise - How To Stay In Motion Without Breathing Problems

Session # 5: Mind, Spirit & Breath - Thinking, Chanting, Prayers As Breathing Exercises

CDs and Downloads

Buteyko Breathing Exercises & Method CD

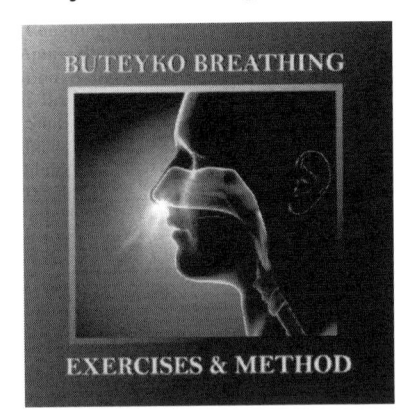

This audio course contains information about K. Buteyko MD-PhD, his discovery and method, breathing and health evaluation as well as breathing exercises. This training course is an easy way to learn about the Buteyko Method and start applying it.

By Thomas Fredricksen

Breathing Normalization Meditations CD

It is easy—listen, enjoy and relax! These guided meditations will help you develop healthier breathing through relaxation and establishing correct breathing patterns. This recording helps stop asthma and anxiety attacks, mouth breathing and various breathing problems. For adults and children.

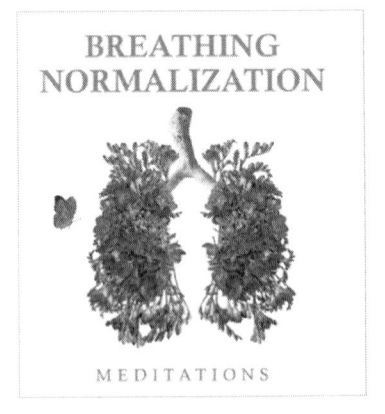

By Sasha Yakovleva

Healing Through Breathing: The Ancient Mantra

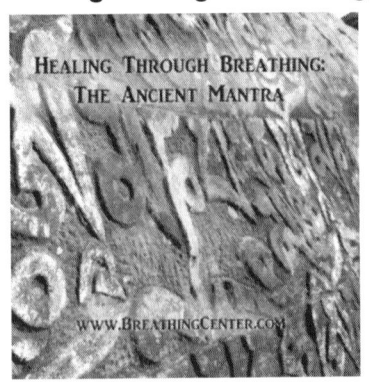

Chanting of Sanskrit mantra, known for its healing qualities. K. Buteyko was the first scientist who discovered that this ancient mantra was capable of improving breathing. This recording is used as breathing training.

Books and Downloads

Adenoids Without Surgery:

Breathing Exercises and Lifestyle Recommendations to Help Children Avoid Adenoidectomy Naturally.

By Sasha Yakovleva

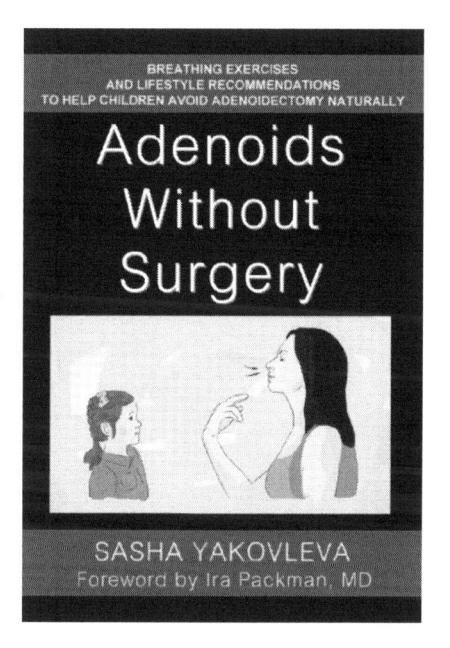

Breathing Exercise Buteyko Logbook

This is a specifically designed journal to record breathing exercises and keep track of breathing improvement.

By Sasha Yakovleva

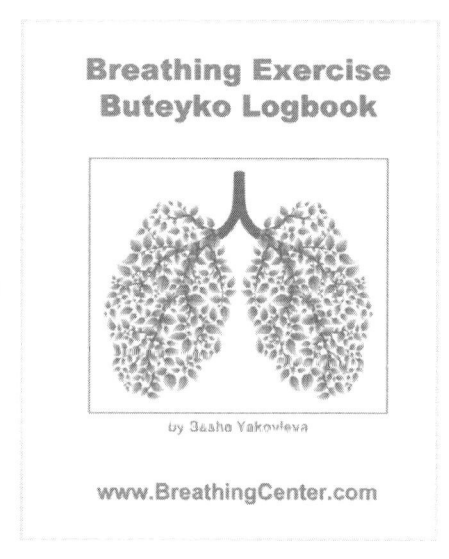

Educational Services Online

Breathing Center offers a variety of educational programs for adults and children. All these programs are available online and can be taken from any location in the world. These courses are individual; however, families, couples or even a small group of friends are welcome to work with a Breathing Normalization Specialist together.

Level 1: Breathing Normalization Training Overcome Health Challenges

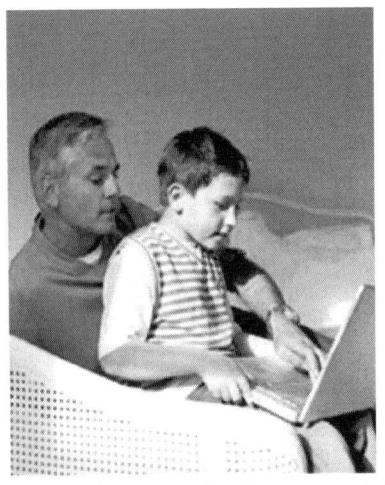

This individual/family training is for adults and children who wish to improve their breathing and health. This program is all-inclusive: it contains everything a person needs to learn and apply the method successfully. It includes weekly online sessions with a Breathing Normalization Specialist, daily support via email, a box of educational materials (DVDs. CDs and books), a box of helpful tools and unlimited support after completion of this program. This is the most effective program for those who would like to tame their asthma or overcome other health challenges. This program takes two months minimum.

Level 2: Breathing Normalization Training
Optimal Health & Longevity

Level 3: Breathing Normalization Training
Learn How to Help Others

Level 4 Breathing Normalization Training:
Start Helping Others

Private Session With A Breathing Normalization Specialist

This service is for anyone that has questions regarding the Breathing Normalization method or Dr. Buteyko's approach. During this session, a Breathing Normalization Specialist answers the student's questions and adjusts the individual program to the student's current needs. You are also welcome to use this type of session to practice guided breathing exercises. Sessions are offered via Skype or in person.

Private Session With Dr. Novozhilov

Online individual consultation with A. Novozhilov MD, the co-founder and Medical Director of Clinica Buteyko in Moscow. This is a unique chance to discuss specifics of Dr. Buteyko's work or your personal application of the method with the true expert.
Simultaneous Russian/English translation is included.

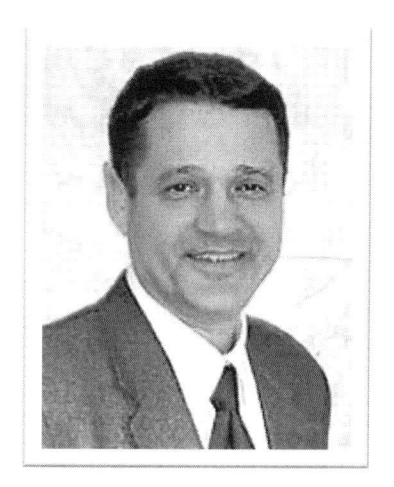

FREE PRELIMINARY CONSULTATION

This consultation will take place via Skype with an Advanced Breathing Normalization Specialist. The Preliminary Consultation is for people considering taking Level 1 Breathing Normalization training. The goal is to help a client (and members of his/her family) evaluate the potential effect of the Breathing Normalization method on their life. This consultation gives the student an opportunity to ask questions. During this 45-minute session, the teacher learns about the client's health history, evaluates their breathing, and briefly explains the theory and application of Buteyko Breathing Normalization, the drug-free and holistic method. For adults and children accompanied by parents.

Afterword

Help Others Learn About Dr. Buteyko's Breathing Normalization

This information has helped thousands of people around the globe overcome various breathing difficulties and hopefully, it will help you as well.

Please feel free to pass this book to your relatives, friends or acquaintances suffering from asthma and various breathing problems or those who are in need of health improvement. We believe that people are entitled to know about a life-saving discovery of Dr. Buteyko and work of Clinica Buteyko Moscow and Breathing Center.

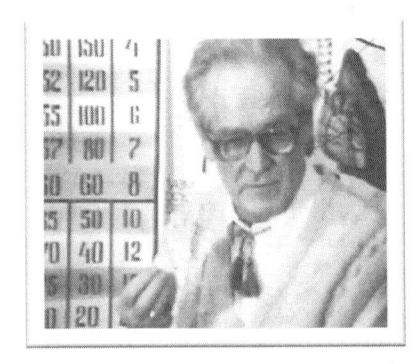

If you purchased this book on one of Amazon's websites, or anywhere, please take a few minutes to write a review and publish it on Amazon. It does not need to be long; even a couple of sentences could be beneficial. This will help others to find the information about Dr. Buteyko's discovery and the Breathing Normalization Method and find the path to tame their asthma.

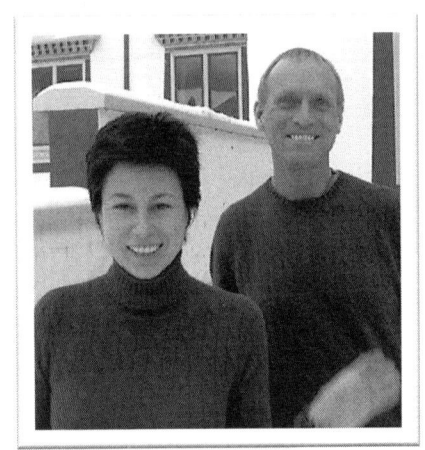

If you have any questions, comments or suggestions, please don't hesitate to contact us at **info@breathingcenter.com**.

In Good Health,
Sasha Yakovleva &
Thomas Fredricksen
Co-founders of
BreathingCenter.com

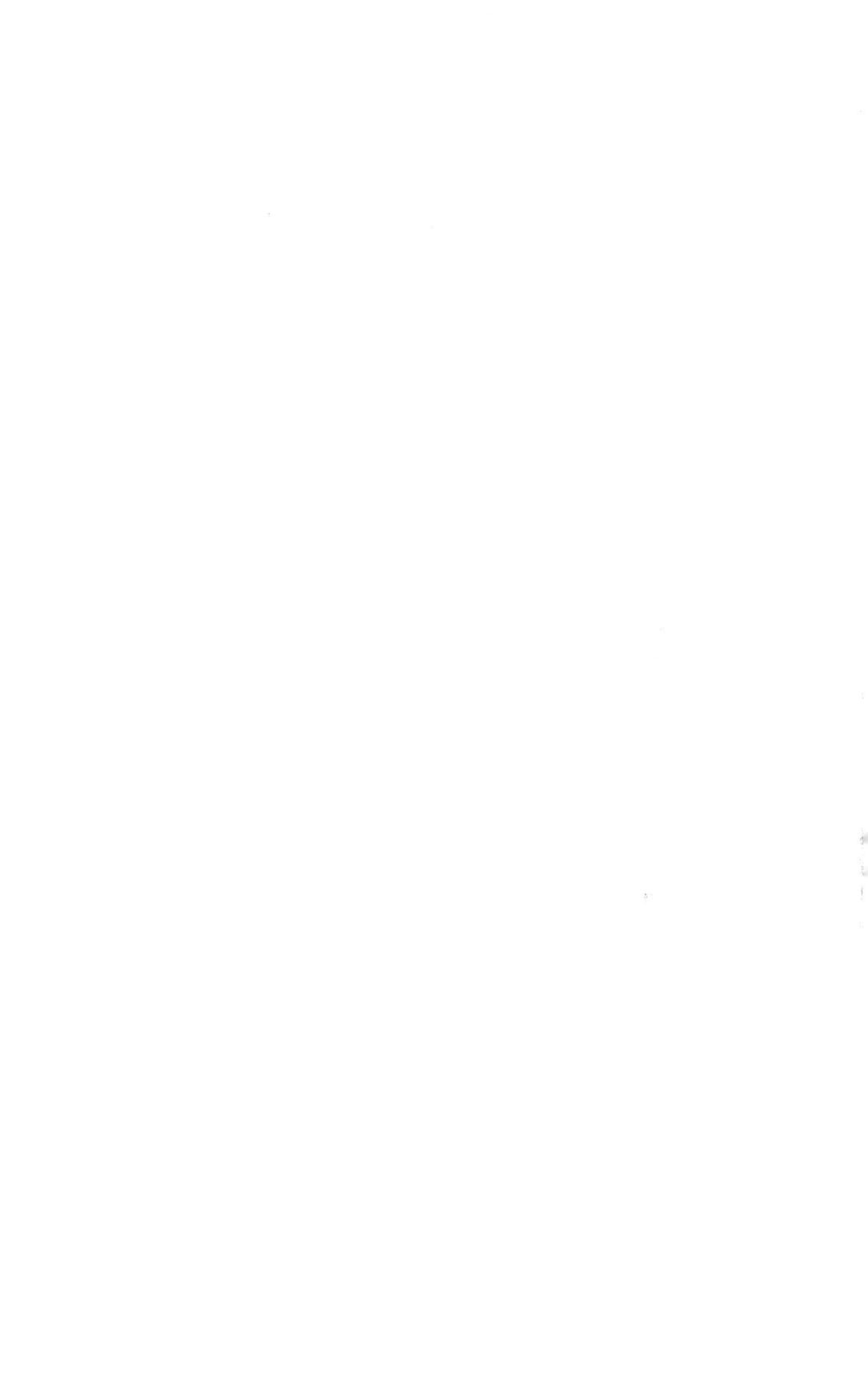